The Polycystic Kidney Mastery Bible
Your Blueprint For Complete Polycystic Kidney Management

Dr. Ankita Kashyap and Prof. Krishna N. Sharma

Published by Virtued Press, 2023.

THE POLYCYSTIC KIDNEY MASTERY BIBLE YOUR BLUEPRINT FOR COMPLETE POLYCYSTIC KIDNEY MANAGEMENT

First edition. November 13, 2023.

ISBN: 979-8223802662

Written by Dr. Ankita Kashyap and Prof. Krishna N. Sharma.

Table of Contents

DISCLAIMER

The information provided in this book is intended for general informational purposes only. The content is not meant to substitute professional medical advice, diagnosis, or treatment. Always consult with a qualified healthcare provider before making any changes to your diabetes management plan or healthcare regimen.

While every effort has been made to ensure the accuracy and completeness of the information presented, the author and publisher do not assume any responsibility for errors, omissions, or potential misinterpretations of the content. Individual responses to diabetes management strategies may vary, and what works for one person might not be suitable for another.

The book does not endorse any specific medical treatments, products, or services. Readers are encouraged to seek guidance from their healthcare providers to determine the most appropriate approaches for their unique medical conditions and needs.

Any external links or resources provided in the book are for convenience and informational purposes only. The author and publisher do not have control over the content or availability of these external sources and do not endorse or guarantee the accuracy of such information.

Readers are advised to exercise caution and use their judgment when applying the information provided in this book to their own situations. The author and publisher disclaim any liability for any direct, indirect, consequential, or other damages arising from the use of this book and its content.

By reading and using this book, readers acknowledge and accept the limitations and inherent risks associated with implementing the strategies, recommendations, and information contained herein. It is always recommended to consult a qualified healthcare professional for personalized medical advice and care.

Introduction

Have you ever imagined what it would be like to have a personal guide with the skills and knowledge required to successfully negotiate the challenging world of managing polycystic kidney disease? Imagine setting out on a quest of discovery, where each step is well thought out and decisions are informed by insights supported by data and workable tactics. That's where your search ends, dear reader. Welcome to Your Comprehensive Guide to Polycystic Kidney Management, The Polycystic Kidney Mastery Bible.

I cordially invite you to embark on a life-changing journey with me as we delve into the complexities of polycystic kidney disease within the pages of this book. My heart and soul have gone into creating a resource that will be your best friend in the quest for holistic health and well-being. I have done this with the unshakable goal of empowering and inspiring others who are dealing with this illness.

You may be confident that every word you read as we go deeper into this adventure has been carefully researched and consulted reliable medical publications and reputable scientific studies. I really think that information is power, and you can take a big step toward taking back control of your life by arming yourself with a thorough awareness of the complexities of polycystic kidney disease.

But have no fear, my friend—this isn't a clinical and boring read. No, instead of being a complex and daunting journey, ours will be one of warmth and compassion as we make our way through the often difficult terrain of managing polycystic kidney disease. You see, my goal in writing this book was to establish a haven of understanding and support rather than just provide medical data and figures. I want to comfort and uplift others with every word I write, like a soft hug in the midst of hardship.

I have made an effort to achieve a healthy balance between the medical and holistic health perspectives throughout our investigation.

By taking into account both modalities, we unearth a wealth of tactics and methods that can coexist in ideal harmony, offering a complete arsenal for your path to wellbeing. I do not cut any corners in my effort to provide you with a wide range of solutions, each customised to meet your specific needs, from traditional medical interventions to alternative and complementary therapies.

However, this book's unwavering commitment to you, the reader, is what really makes it unique. I am aware that every person with polycystic kidney disease is unique and has complex effects. I have therefore taken great care to provide individualised programmes and self-help methods, making sure that each suggestion fits well into the overall picture of your life. I'm here to help you at every stage of your journey, regardless of how long you've been dealing with polycystic kidney disease.

Let us keep in mind that we are not alone as we go out on this journey of empowerment and education. You will find a thriving community of people who understand your struggles, goals, and dreams within the pages of this book. As a group, we will compose a symphony of resiliency and victory, with every note adding to the grand totality of healing and wellbeing.

I now extend an invitation to you, my dear reader, to join me on this incredible journey. Let's explore the mysteries surrounding the treatment of polycystic kidney disease—not as a hardship to be endured, but as a chance to develop, become knowledgeable, and prosper. You have the ability to take back your life if you use The Polycystic Kidney Mastery Bible as your guide. Are you prepared to go on this life-changing adventure? I'll start now.

Chapter 1: Understanding Polycystic Kidney Disease

Genetic Factors in Polycystic Kidney Disease

A hereditary condition known as polycystic kidney disease (PKD) is typified by the development of many kidney cysts. Millions of people are impacted globally, and if addressed, it can result in serious renal dysfunction and failure. Comprehending the genetic elements that contribute to Parkinson's disease (PKD) is crucial for precise diagnosis, effective disease management, and the creation of focused treatment strategies.

As a physician and health and wellness coach, I have devoted my professional life to assisting people with Parkinson's disease (PKD) in comprehending and navigating the intricacies of this illness. My team and I, comprising a varied group of medical professionals, offer comprehensive care that attends to the mental, emotional, and physical elements of managing Parkinson's disease.

Mutations in particular genes, which are essential for the growth and operation of the kidneys, result in PKD. Gene mutations are the primary cause of the two main forms of PKD, autosomal recessive PKD (ARPKD) and autosomal dominant PKD (ADPKD).

Mutations in the PKD1 or PKD2 gene generate ADPKD, the most prevalent kind of PKD. These genes produce proteins that control kidney cell growth and division as well as the development of cilia, which are microscopic hair-like projections on the cells. Cyst development results from aberrant cell proliferation caused by mutations in these genes.

ADPKD inherits according to an autosomal dominant pattern. This indicates that there is a 50% probability of inheriting the mutant gene and getting ADPKD if one parent has the condition. To ascertain their risk and take the necessary action for early intervention, anyone with a family history of ADPKD should consider genetic testing.

Conversely, while less prevalent than ADPKD, ARPKD is associated with a higher chance of kidney failure in early childhood and more severe symptoms. The PKHD1 gene, which codes for the protein fibrocystin, is mutated in ARPKD. The proper growth and operation of the kidneys depend on this protein.

Because ARPKD has an autosomal recessive inheritance pattern, a child cannot acquire the disease unless both parents have a copy of the defective gene. Genetic counselling is advised in families where there is a known history of ARPKD in order to determine the risk and direct family planning.

Not only has the diagnosis of Parkinson's disease (PKD) been transformed by the discovery of its genetic basis, but tailored treatments have also become possible. Particular medications that specifically target the biochemical pathways impacted by the genetic alterations in PKD have been developed by researchers.

For example, drugs that precisely block the action of specific proteins encoded by the mutant genes are now available for ADPKD. These medications, sometimes referred to as vasopressin receptor antagonists, aid in maintaining renal function and slowing the formation of cysts.

Research on ARPKD has concentrated on creating medications that can make the mutant protein, fibrocystin, functional again. Promising progress has been made with gene therapy and tailored pharmaceutical methods, while more study is required.

For those with a family history of the condition, the identification and comprehension of the genetic components causing Parkinson's disease have important ramifications. Even before symptoms appear, genetic testing can now be used to identify whether a person has inherited the faulty gene. Proactive management and the adoption of lifestyle changes that can halt the advancement of the disease are made possible by early diagnosis.

Furthermore, because PKD is inherited, affected individuals may face emotional and psychological difficulties. It can be debilitating to realise that their illness is hereditary and may impact future generations. For this reason, psychological assistance and counselling are essential parts of the comprehensive care that PKD patients and their families get.

In conclusion, the development, diagnosis, and available treatments of polycystic kidney disease are significantly influenced by the genetic elements that underlie the condition. Targeted therapies, genetic testing, and proactive management techniques are made possible by an understanding of the particular genes and inheritance patterns linked to Parkinson's disease (PKD). People with Parkinson's disease (PKD) can manage their hereditary risk and maximise their general well-being by taking a complete and holistic approach.

Symptoms and Diagnosis of Polycystic Kidney Disease

I have treated many patients with polycystic kidney disease in my capacity as a medical doctor who specialises in holistic healthcare (PKD). I now have a better understanding of the range of symptoms that people with Parkinson's disease (PKD) may encounter. I'll go over the typical symptoms you should be aware of in this subchapter, along with the diagnostic techniques used to determine whether PKD is present.

Abdominal pain is one of the main signs of Parkinson's disease. Kidney cyst formation is frequently the cause of this pain. These cysts are sacs filled with fluid that can form in the kidneys and enlarge over time. Growing cysts may put pressure on the tissues and organs nearby, causing pain and discomfort. Abdominal discomfort associated with Parkinson's disease (PKD) can be either dull and aching or severe and stabbing. Each person will experience discomfort differently, and it could get worse after eating a heavy meal or during physical exertion.

An additional typical PKD symptom is elevated blood pressure. Blood pressure might rise as a result of the kidneys' malfunctioning normally, which can be caused by cysts. For those who have PKD, high blood pressure is a serious concern because it can exacerbate the disease's course and cause additional kidney damage. People with PKD should take the required precautions to control their blood pressure and monitor it on a regular basis.

Another typical PKD symptom is urinary issues. Renal cyst formation can impede the regular flow of urine, resulting in problems like blood in the urine, difficulty urinating, or frequent urination. Hematuria, or the presence of blood in the urine, can be concerning and has to be treated very away. Urinary issues can, however, also indicate other medical disorders, so getting a proper diagnosis from a healthcare provider is essential.

A variety of diagnostic techniques are employed to determine the severity and establish the existence of PKD. An ultrasound is one of the most common imaging examinations performed. High-frequency sound waves are used in ultrasound to produce images of the kidneys and find cysts. Through this non-invasive treatment, physicians can see the quantity and size of kidney cysts.

Certain situations may need the use of additional imaging tests, such as magnetic resonance imaging (MRI) or computed tomography (CT) scans (MRI). These examinations offer more precise pictures of the kidneys and can be used to gauge how big the cyst has gotten. In contrast to an MRI, which creates comprehensive images of the body's internal components using radio waves and magnetic fields, a CT scan entails capturing several X-ray images from different angles.

Another vital diagnosis method for Parkinson's disease is genetic testing. Since PKD is a hereditary condition, it can be inherited from either or both parents. Genetic testing can identify particular genes linked to Parkinson's disease (PKD) and ascertain whether a given person carries a mutation in these genes. Those who have a family history of Parkinson's disease (PKD) or who intend to become parents and would like to know their likelihood of passing the illness on to their children may find this test helpful.

Patients with PKD must have regular kidney function monitoring in addition to these diagnostic tests. Tests on blood are part of this to evaluate kidney function and look for variations in blood chemistry. Healthcare providers can use these tests to inform treatment decisions by determining the patient's PKD stage.

In summary, comprehensive awareness of PKD symptoms and proper diagnosis techniques are essential for managing the illness effectively. Urinary issues, elevated blood pressure, and abdominal pain are prominent signs of Parkinson's disease (PKD) that people should be aware of. Diagnostic techniques include MRIs, CT scans, ultrasounds, and genetic testing can assist determine the degree and presence of Parkinson's disease (PKD). Effective management of Parkinson's disease (PKD) also requires routine renal function monitoring. People with Parkinson's disease (PKD) can improve their quality of life and overall health by quickly recognising and treating these symptoms.

Risk Factors for Polycystic Kidney Disease

Age is a major risk factor for Parkinson's disease. Studies have indicated that the occurrence of this disorder rises with age. The symptoms of Parkinson's disease (PKD) usually appear in maturity, particularly in the 30s and 40s. Sometimes people don't show any symptoms until they're in their fifties or sixties. This evolution over time emphasises how crucial routine examinations and screenings are, especially as people age. Prognosis can be greatly enhanced by early detection, which also makes timely management and intervention possible.

Gender is an additional risk factor that cannot be disregarded. Research has repeatedly demonstrated that the effects of PKD are nearly comparable in men and women. Nonetheless, there can be certain gender-specific factors to take into account. For example, studies have revealed that women are more likely than men to have larger cysts and to have frequent and severe symptoms. These variations could be attributed to hormonal shifts that occur during menstruation, pregnancy, and menopause. Women must collaborate closely with their healthcare providers to develop appropriate management measures and be aware of these potential implications.

An important factor in the development of PKD is family history. Because PKD is a hereditary disorder, people who have a family history of the illness are more likely to get it themselves. Autosomal dominant PKD (ADPKD) and autosomal recessive PKD are the two main forms of PKD (ARPKD). The most prevalent kind, ADPKD, is usually inherited from one affected parent. In contrast, ARPKD is uncommon and typically manifests in early childhood or infancy. Regular screenings and consultation with a healthcare provider are imperative for individuals who have a close family member, such as a parent or sibling, with Parkinson's disease (PKD) to discuss preventive strategies.

Hypertension, or high blood pressure, is a risk factor that is strongly linked to Parkinson's disease (PKD). In actuality, hypertension is a frequent side effect of this illness in addition to being a risk factor. The normal structure and function of the kidneys are disrupted when cysts grow in this essential organ. This disturbance may cause blood pressure to rise, which could further harm the kidneys. This leads to a vicious cycle in which hypertension aggravates kidney injury, and kidney damage exacerbates hypertension. People who have Parkinson's kidney disease (PKD) must constantly check their blood pressure and manage it with medicine and lifestyle changes.

A few lifestyle decisions can also affect how PKD develops and is managed. For example, it has been determined that smoking increases the risk of kidney disease, including PKD. Researchers have shown that smoking can exacerbate renal function in people with PKD and hasten the development of cysts. Consequently, it is strongly advised that smokers who are at risk or have already been diagnosed with PKD give up. Additionally, kidney health can benefit from keeping a healthy weight and getting regular exercise. These changes in lifestyle can help control blood pressure, lessen the burden on the kidneys, and enhance the quality of life for those who have peripheral kidney disease (PKD).

In conclusion, people can manage their health more proactively by being aware of and comprehending the risk factors connected to polycystic kidney disease. A person's age, gender, family history, high blood pressure, and lifestyle choices can all raise their risk of developing peripheral vascular disease (PKD). Through consistent blood pressure monitoring, tests, lifestyle modifications, and close collaboration with healthcare providers, individuals can substantially mitigate their chance of getting this chronic illness or efficiently manage it in the event of a diagnosis. Keep in mind that information is empowering when it comes to preserving renal health at its best and general wellbeing.

Types of Polycystic Kidney Disease

1. Autosomal Dominant PKD (ADPKD):

About 90% of all cases of PKD are Autosomal Dominant PKD, which is the most prevalent type of the disease. Kidney cysts develop as a result of a mutation in the PKD1 or PKD2 gene, which causes ADPKD. This genetic abnormality causes the kidneys' tubules to form abnormally, which eventually causes cysts to get larger.

The symptoms of ADPKD normally appear in adults, mainly between the ages of 30 and 40, however they can occasionally appear earlier or later. Even among members of the same family line, there can be significant individual variation in the clinical characteristics of ADPKD. Hematuria (blood in the urine), kidney stones, hypertension, frequent urinary tract infections (UTIs), and flank pain are common symptoms. The kidneys gradually lose their ability to function normally as the cysts get bigger and multiply, which can eventually result in end-stage renal disease (ESRD) or chronic kidney disease (CKD).

The inheritance pattern of ADPKD is a crucial feature. With a 50% risk of transmission, ADPKD is an autosomal dominant condition that can be handed down from one generation to the next. This indicates that each child has a 50% probability of inheriting the mutant gene and getting ADPKD if one or both parents have the disorder. When it comes to family planning, genetic testing can assist identify the presence of the mutation even before symptoms appear.

2. Autosomal Recessive PKD (ARPKD):

Autosomal Recessive PKD, which makes up only 10% of all PKD cases, is far less frequent than ADPKD. While the underlying processes of ARPKD are distinct from those of ADPKD, both disorders are caused by mutations in the PKHD1 gene and result in comparable cyst formation.

ARPKD is usually detected in infancy or early childhood, unlike ADPKD. Infants affected with this condition may exhibit a variety of symptoms, such as poor lung development, high blood pressure, abnormalities of the urinary tract, and enlarged kidneys (hepatosplenomegaly). In addition to structural liver issues such hepatic fibrosis or Caroli disease, infants with ARPKD may also experience other health complications.

The autosomal recessive mode of inheritance is observed in ARPKD. This indicates that for a child to inherit the ailment, both parents must have a copy of the defective gene. Each child has a 25% chance of inheriting two copies of the mutant gene, which causes ARPKD, if both parents are carriers. Families having a history of ARPKD must have genetic counselling and testing in order to fully comprehend the risk and make decisions.

Prevalence of PKD in different populations:

PKD affects individuals from a wide range of ethnic backgrounds and is a global health concern. However, due to genetic and environmental variables, the prevalence of Parkinson's disease (PKD) can range among various cultures.

All racial and ethnic groupings have equal prevalence rates of ADPKD. But compared to other populations, some have a higher prevalence than others, such as those of European heritage. Research indicates that between one in five hundred and one thousand people of European ancestry suffer from ADPKD. Conversely, people of Asian or African origin typically have a reduced frequency of ADPKD.

In contrast, there are variations in the prevalence of ARPKD according to racial and ethnic background. Research has indicated that people of African or African-American heritage are more likely to have ARPKD, which is thought to affect 1 in 20,000 live births. Individuals with European or Asian heritage typically have a lower prevalence, estimated at 1 in 40,000 to 1 in 50,000. These differences in prevalence emphasise how critical it is to comprehend the hereditary and environmental elements that contribute to PKD development in various groups.

To sum up, it is essential to comprehend the many forms of polycystic kidney disease in order to provide precise diagnosis, treatment, and genetic counselling. The most prevalent type, known as autosomal dominant Parkinson's disease (ADPKD), usually manifests in adulthood and is inherited in an autosomal dominant manner. On the other hand, autosomal recessive Parkinson's disease (ARPKD) is less frequent, typically detected in early childhood or infancy, and has an autosomal recessive inheritance pattern. Both varieties can have varying prevalences in various groups; people of European origin are typically more likely to have ADPKD, while those of varying racial and ethnic backgrounds are more likely to have ARPKD. A thorough grasp of these varieties and their frequency will enable us to better customise our management strategy for polycystic kidney disease and give those who suffer from the illness more specialised medical care.

Chapter 2: Medical Management of Polycystic Kidney Disease

Medications for Polycystic Kidney Disease

Medication is a vital part of controlling Polycystic Kidney Disease (PKD) because it helps to both relieve symptoms and slow down the disease's progression. While medicine cannot treat Parkinson's disease (PKD) on its own, it can greatly enhance a patient's quality of life when taken in conjunction with other treatment methods and lifestyle changes.

The kind of medicine provided for Parkinson's disease (PKD) is determined by a number of variables, including the patient's preferences, the severity and stage of the disease, and the existence of complications. I treat PKD patients holistically, taking into account their individual needs, as a medical doctor with a focus on holistic therapy. We are able to offer a comprehensive approach to PKD management because my team of experts consists of experts from various sectors related to health and wellbeing.

A thorough grasp of the drugs frequently used in PKD therapy is essential to developing an efficient treatment plan. Let's examine these drugs' specifics, including how they work, any possible adverse effects, and how to customise them to a patient's needs.

1. Angiotensin-Converting Enzyme (ACE) Inhibitors:

ACE inhibitors are frequently prescribed drugs that assist PKD patients in controlling their blood pressure. They accomplish this by preventing the enzyme that produces the hormone angiotensin II, which narrows blood vessels and raises blood pressure, from doing its job. ACE inhibitors can help delay the progression of kidney impairment in PKD by lowering blood pressure. ACE inhibitors that are frequently administered include Ramipril, Enalapril, and Lisinopril. Hypotension, lightheadedness, and a dry cough are possible adverse effects.

2. Angiotensin II Receptor Blockers (ARBs):

Like ACE inhibitors, angiotensin II's activities are blocked by ARBs, which likewise aid in blood pressure regulation. They function at a distinct stage of the hormone cascade, though. When ACE inhibitors cause negative effects in a patient, ARBs are frequently recommended as a substitute. ARBs that are frequently prescribed include Irbesartan, Valsartan, and Losartan. Low blood pressure, dizziness, and an elevated risk of excessive potassium levels are possible side effects.

3. Diuretics:

Diuretics, commonly referred to as "water pills," are drugs that cause the body to produce more pee, which helps eliminate extra fluid. Patients with PKD who have edoema and fluid retention are frequently administered them. Furosemide is the diuretic that is prescribed for PKD the most frequently. Frequent urination, electrolyte imbalances, and dehydration are possible side effects.

4. Pain Medications:

Since kidney enlargement or cyst rupture frequently cause discomfort in patients, pain management is a crucial part of treating Parkinson's disease (PKD). Ibuprofen and Naproxen are two examples of non-steroidal anti-inflammatory medicines (NSAIDs) that are frequently used for mild to moderate pain. But it's crucial to utilise these drugs carefully since if taken in excess or for an extended length of time, they may harm the kidneys. Stronger painkillers, such opioids, may occasionally be recommended for extremely severe pain. Because of the possibility of dependence and other negative effects, these drugs should only be taken under the strict guidance of a physician.

5. Antibiotics:

Patients with Parkinson's disease (PKD) are more likely to experience urinary tract infections (UTIs) because to kidney abnormalities and perhaps bacterial cysts. Treating UTIs as soon as possible is essential to avoiding problems. PKD patients are frequently taken antibiotics, such as trimethoprim-sulfamethoxazole and ciprofloxacin, to treat UTIs. To guarantee efficient treatment, it's critical to adhere to the recommended antibiotic course and finish it entirely.

These are but a handful of the drugs that are frequently prescribed for the treatment of Parkinson's disease. As a health and wellness coach, I think it's critical to have personalised treatment programmes that are made to meet the specific requirements of every patient. When prescribing drugs, this entails taking into account many characteristics like general health, kidney function, and possible drug interactions. To guarantee the safe and efficient use of drugs, constant collaboration with a healthcare team that specialises in PKD management is essential.

The management of Parkinson's disease (PKD) involves not only medication but also lifestyle adjustments and other therapeutic techniques. This include eating a kidney-friendly diet, exercising frequently, controlling stress, abstaining from smoking, and consuming little or no alcohol. Acupuncture, yoga, and meditation are examples of complementary therapies that may be helpful in controlling symptoms and enhancing general wellbeing.

In summary, drugs constitute a crucial component in treating Parkinson's disease (PKD), but they are not a stand-alone treatment. For the disease to be effectively managed, a comprehensive strategy that incorporates medication along with lifestyle changes, complementary therapies, and routine monitoring is necessary. In my dual roles as a physician and a health and wellness coach, I work hard to give my patients comprehensive care with the goal of enhancing their quality of life and giving them the tools they need to take control of their health. By working together, we may successfully traverse the complexity of Parkinson's disease (PKD) and create individualised treatment plans that allow patients to fully enjoy life.

Surgical Interventions for Polycystic Kidney Disease

A surgical treatment called cyst decortication, or cyst fenestration, entails puncturing and emptying specific kidney cysts. Patients with symptomatic cysts that cause pain, infection, or urinary blockage are frequently the ones who have this operation. Cyst decortication involves the surgeon making tiny incisions in the afflicted areas and using laparoscopic tools to remove the cyst fluid. This can stop the cyst from growing further and offer instant symptom relief. It's crucial to understand that cyst decortication does not treat Parkinson's disease (PKD) or stop the formation of new cysts. It's a palliative procedure designed to reduce symptoms and enhance quality of life.

On the other side, a nephrectomy entails removing one or both kidneys. Patients with end-stage renal disease (ESRD) who have significantly enlarged kidneys that are resulting in problems like discomfort, infection, or hypertension are usually the only ones eligible for this operation. Both open surgery and laparoscopic methods can be used to perform a nephrectomy, depending on the patient's general condition and the severity of the disease. Nephrectomy may occasionally be taken into consideration as a prophylactic strategy in patients whose PKD is advancing quickly or in those who are highly susceptible to problems. A nephrectomy is a significant surgery that permanently removes the kidneys, necessitating dialysis or a kidney transplant for the patient to survive, therefore it's crucial to carefully consider the risks and advantages.

The most successful course of treatment for patients with PKD-related ESRD is kidney transplantation. It entails the surgical implantation of a donor kidney, either living or deceased, into the body of the recipient. For PKD patients with ESRD, kidney transplantation provides the greatest long-term results in terms of survival and quality of life. A successful kidney transplant can also return normal kidney function and remove the requirement for dialysis. It is crucial to remember that a kidney transplant does not treat Parkinson's disease (PKD) because the patient's remaining kidney or kidneys may still develop cysts. Therefore, in order to guarantee early detection and control of any potential problems, transplant recipients must have continuous monitoring and follow-up care.

It is important to consider carefully before deciding to get surgery for Parkinson's disease. Careful assessment of the patient's overall health, the course of the disease, and their unique situation is necessary. A comprehensive pre-operative evaluation is carried out before every surgical treatment in order to determine whether the patient is a good candidate for surgery as well as to identify any possible risks or contraindications.

Pre-operative assessment consists of a physical examination, a thorough medical history, and several diagnostic procedures. Blood tests to measure kidney function, imaging tests (CT or ultrasound) to determine the position and size of cysts, and genetic testing to confirm the diagnosis of PKD and find any related gene alterations are a few examples of these.

It is crucial to take into account the patient's coping mechanisms and psychological health in addition to these routine evaluations. Surgical interventions can be emotionally taxing, and PKD can have a substantial negative influence on a patient's mental health and quality of life. In order to make sure that patients are well-prepared and have reasonable expectations regarding the surgical procedures and their possible consequences, psychological evaluation and counselling may be helpful.

Following the determination that the patient is a good candidate for surgery, the surgeon will go over the possible advantages and disadvantages of each surgical procedure and collaborate with the patient to create a personalised treatment plan. Surgical interventions may be combined in this strategy based on the unique demands and circumstances of the patient.

It is crucial to remember that surgical procedures carry some dangers even if they can reduce symptoms and enhance quality of life. Nephrectomy and cyst decortication may result in haemorrhage, infection, harm to neighbouring organs, and hernia development. Risks associated with kidney transplantation include infection, rejection of the donated organ, and adverse effects from immunosuppressive drugs.

It is essential to select skilled surgeons who specialise in PKD surgery and to closely adhere to all pre- and post-operative instructions in order to reduce these risks and guarantee the best results. Furthermore, patients ought to take an active role in their own care, making lifestyle changes and adhering to therapy and drug regimens in order to maximise their general health and well-being.

In summary, surgical procedures are essential to the therapy of Parkinson's disease (PKD) because they alleviate symptoms, enhance quality of life, and increase survival times for individuals with end-stage renal disease (ESRD). Nephrectomy, kidney transplantation, and cyst decortication are all feasible treatments that need to be carefully evaluated in light of the specifics of each patient and the course of their illness. But it's crucial to keep in mind that PKD cannot be cured by surgery, and that ongoing monitoring and follow-up treatment are necessary to identify and treat any potential consequences. Patients with PKD can maximise their treatment outcomes and reach a greater degree of illness mastery by cooperating with a multidisciplinary team of medical specialists, comprising surgeons, nephrologists, and mental health specialists.

Dialysis and Polycystic Kidney Disease

Let's start by going over the fundamentals of dialysis. When the kidneys are unable to effectively eliminate waste materials, extra fluid, and poisons from the body, dialysis is a medical technique that can help. Dialysis is required in the case of PKD when the kidneys' overall function declines due to the formation and expansion of kidney cysts. It is a crucial kind of treatment for those with Parkinson's disease, particularly when the illness is more advanced.

Hemodialysis:

The most popular type of dialysis is hemodialysis, which is normally carried out at a facility dedicated to this type of treatment. The patient's blood is removed from the body during hemodialysis via a vascular access point, such as a catheter or an arteriovenous fistula. After that, the blood passes through a dialyzer, a device that functions as an artificial kidney by removing waste and extra fluid from the blood before reintroducing the cleansed blood into the body.

The ability of hemodialysis to effectively and efficiently remove toxins and waste products contributes to the maintenance of a relatively stable internal environment, which is one of its key benefits. It can be done sporadically, for a few hours each session, usually three times a week. This permits patients to maintain some degree of schedule flexibility and to carry out their regular activities.

Nevertheless, hemodialysis has its limitations as well. First of all, it necessitates frequent trips to a dialysis facility, which can be inconvenient for patients and time-consuming. Second, to guarantee a smooth blood flow during dialysis, the vascular access point—such as an arteriovenous fistula or catheter—must be established and maintained appropriately. It is possible for complications like infections or clotting to occur, necessitating continuing observation and possible therapies. Finally, the decreased clearance capacity of the kidneys during hemodialysis necessitates the implementation of dietary and fluid restrictions, which can be difficult for certain patients to follow.

Peritoneal Dialysis:

An alternate form of dialysis that can be done at home and gives patients some degree of treatment autonomy is peritoneal dialysis. Peritoneal dialysis, as contrast to hemodialysis, uses the peritoneal membrane—a lining found inside the abdomen—as a natural filter to remove waste products.

A catheter is surgically placed into the belly to facilitate the infusion and outflow of dialysate, a unique dialysis solution, during peritoneal dialysis. After being inserted into the abdominal cavity and held there for a while—usually a few hours—the dialysate is removed along with waste materials and extra fluid. An exchange can be carried out manually or with the assistance of a device called a cycler.

The flexibility that peritoneal dialysis provides is one of its main benefits. Patients have more control over their treatment plan when they are able to complete exchanges at their place of employment, home, or while travelling. Furthermore, peritoneal dialysis may be superior to hemodialysis in terms of blood pressure control and preservation of residual kidney function.

Peritoneal dialysis can have certain drawbacks, though. First of all, in order to reduce the danger of infection, a certain amount of dedication and careful sterile procedure adherence are required throughout exchanges. Second, some individuals may find it difficult to go through the exchange procedure several times a day. Finally, peritoneal dialysis may not be appropriate for some metabolic abnormalities, such as elevated blood sugar in diabetic patients or obesity.

In summary, dialysis is essential for the treatment of polycystic kidney disease, especially in its latter stages when renal function is substantially impaired. The two primary forms of dialysis utilised for individuals with PKD are hemodialysis and peritoneal dialysis, each with unique benefits and drawbacks. Dialysis is selected based on the specific needs and preferences of each patient, taking into account medical eligibility, lifestyle, and preferences.

In my capacity as a physician and health and wellness coach, I stress the value of a multidisciplinary approach to the treatment of Parkinson's disease. Comprehensive care includes not only dialysis but also nutritional planning, lifestyle adjustments, and psychological support. We give patients the tools they need to manage their journey with PKD by focusing not just on the physical elements but also on their emotional and mental well-being, thanks to my team of professionals from a variety of health and wellness sectors.

We give patients the tools they need to control their Parkinson's disease completely by providing them with information and comprehension. In order to ensure that every patient's journey with PKD is greeted with compassion, resilience, and a holistic approach to treatment, we work together to achieve optimal health and quality of life.

The Role of Healthcare Professionals in Polycystic Kidney Disease Management

The primary medical specialists involved in the management of Parkinson's kidney disease are nephrologists. They are very knowledgeable about the intricacies of PKD and specialise in the diagnosis and treatment of renal problems. Nephrologists are essential in tracking the course of the illness, controlling symptoms, and carrying out recommended treatment regimens. They are in charge of monitoring blood pressure and renal health, doing routine screenings, and evaluating kidney function. They can assist detect potential issues and create plans to deal with them by keeping a careful eye on these variables.

Urologists are crucial to the treatment of Parkinson's disease (PKD). Diagnosis and treatment of urinary tract problems, especially kidney disorders, is their area of expertise. Urologists specialise in treating big cysts that might impair kidney function or cause pain in patients with Parkinson's disease (PKD). They might carry out a range of procedures, like cyst drainage or writing prescriptions for painkillers. Additionally, urologists are essential in the management of PKD consequences such kidney stones and urinary tract infections. Their knowledge is crucial for guaranteeing the best possible kidney health and for giving PKD patients thorough care.

Additionally, genetic counsellors are quite helpful in managing Parkinson's disease. They are experts in the field of genetics and offer assistance and support to people with genetic illnesses as well as their families. Hereditary counsellors are essential in helping patients and their families understand the genetic component of Parkinson's disease (PKD). They support people in learning about the patterns of PKD inheritance, determining how likely they are to pass the disease on to future generations, and investigating family planning alternatives.

Additionally, genetic counsellors help patients deal with the psychological effects of the disease and its emotional toll. In order to give patients the authority to make decisions about their health and the health of their future generations, their engagement is crucial.

Patients with Parkinson's disease may also profit from the knowledge of other medical specialists, including psychologists, physical therapists, and dieticians. Dieticians can offer invaluable advice in creating the best diet plan for individuals with Parkinson's disease (PKD), taking into account the condition's dietary restrictions as well as the patients' particular nutritional requirements. Additionally, they can support patients in adopting appropriate lifestyle choices that may halt the disease's course and enhance general health. Psychologists can provide therapy and support to individuals with Parkinson's disease (PKD) who may be in substantial emotional distress or who are having difficulty adjusting to the changes and difficulties brought on by the illness. Psychological therapies have the potential to improve patients' quality of life, assist in the development of coping mechanisms, and improve overall health outcomes. Physical therapists can help people with Parkinson's disease (PKD) stay physically fit, control their pain, and increase their range of motion. They are able to design personalised training regimens that consider the special requirements and constraints of each patient.

For PKD patients to receive complete care, various healthcare professionals must coordinate and collaborate with one another. Patients are guaranteed to receive tailored, integrated care that takes into account their particular requirements and difficulties when a multidisciplinary approach is used. Healthcare providers can create a comprehensive strategy that addresses all facets of managing Parkinson's disease (PKD), including medical, genetic, dietary, psychological, and physical factors, by working together and communicating on a regular basis. For PKD patients, an all-encompassing strategy may lead to better results and an enhanced quality of life.

In summary, a multidisciplinary approach is necessary for the care of Parkinson's disease (PKD), with major roles being played by nephrologists, urologists, genetic counsellors, dieticians, psychologists, and physical therapists. In order to provide PKD patients with complete care, healthcare professionals must collaborate with one another. Each brings a unique set of skills and knowledge to the table. Together, they can handle the various facets of the illness and give patients the best treatment available. In my capacity as a physician and health and wellness coach, I fervently support a multidisciplinary team approach to PKD management and a comprehensive approach to healthcare.

Chapter 3: Holistic Approaches to Polycystic Kidney Disease Management

Lifestyle Modifications for Polycystic Kidney Disease

As everyone knows, exercise is essential to preserving general health and wellbeing. However, did you know that managing PKD can also benefit greatly from regular exercise? It has been demonstrated that physical activity improves immunological response, blood circulation, and cardiovascular health. Additionally, it can lower the chance of developing issues associated to kidney disease and help control blood pressure.

Finding enjoyable activities that fit your physical capabilities is crucial when it comes to fitness. It's crucial to remember that not every exercise is appropriate for people with Parkinson's disease. Running and jumping are examples of high-impact exercises that should be avoided since they put additional strain on the kidneys. Rather, choose low-impact workouts like yoga, cycling, swimming, or strolling. These exercises are easy to adapt to your fitness level and have low impact on the joints.

It's also a good idea to speak with your medical team before beginning any new fitness programme. Personalized recommendations and counsel tailored to your unique health needs and restrictions can be given by them.

Keeping up a healthy diet is essential for treating Parkinson's disease (PKD), along with consistent exercise. A diet high in nutrients helps lower inflammation, control blood pressure, and maintain kidney function. Dietary recommendations that are especially helpful for people with PKD include:

1. Limit sodium intake: Elevated blood pressure and fluid retention brought on by high salt levels might further tax the kidneys. A daily intake of fewer than 2,300 mg of salt is advised. Watch out for hidden salt sources such sauces, canned soups, and processed foods.

2. Opt for low-protein foods: Kidney strain can result from consuming too much protein. Selecting protein from lean sources, such fish, chicken, tofu, and beans, will lessen the strain on your kidneys. Aim for a moderate protein consumption; to find the ideal quantity for your needs, speak with a trained dietitian.

3. Increase fruits and vegetables: Antioxidants, vitamins, and minerals that are vital for overall health can be found in plenty in fruits and vegetables. They support normal blood pressure levels and are low in salt. Make it a point to include a range of vibrant fruits and veggies in your daily diet.

4. Stay hydrated: It's essential to drink enough water to keep your kidneys healthy. It aids in the body's removal of waste materials and poisons. Try to consume eight glasses of water or more each day if your doctor recommends it. Alcohol and sugary drinks should not be consumed in excess as they might cause the body to become dehydrated.

A balanced diet, regular exercise, and stress management are all essential to the comprehensive care of Parkinson's disease. Stress hormones are released as a result of the stress reaction, and this can be harmful to kidney function. For this reason, incorporating stress-reduction strategies into your daily routine is essential to preserving kidney health at its best.

There are numerous techniques and practices that you can incorporate into your daily life to help manage stress. Some effective stress-reduction strategies include:

1. Mindfulness and meditation: Stress can be decreased and the mind can become more at ease by setting aside a short amount of time each day to practise mindfulness or meditation. Pay attention to your breathing while objectively observing your thoughts. This exercise can support the development of inner serenity and tranquilly.

2. Physical activity: Regular physical activity improves mental and bodily health in addition to physical health. Endorphins, sometimes

referred to as "feel-good" hormones, are released when you exercise and can help reduce stress and elevate your mood.

3. Relaxation techniques: Stress can be decreased and a state of relaxation can be induced by incorporating relaxation techniques such progressive muscle relaxation, guided imagery, and deep breathing exercises. Choose a method that feels right for you and use it often.

4. Social support: Creating a network of friends, family, or support groups can help you deal with the difficulties of having PKD. Stress can be much reduced and emotional support can be greatly increased by talking to someone about your worries and experiences.

And last, keeping your kidneys healthy requires drinking enough water. Getting adequate fluids aids in the body's removal of waste materials and helps to prevent kidney stones from forming. Water is the ideal beverage to stay hydrated because sugar-filled beverages and high caffeine content might harm the kidneys. Try to consume eight glasses of water or more each day if your doctor advises you to.

In summary, changing one's lifestyle is essential to manage polycystic kidney disease successfully. Important elements of a comprehensive strategy for managing Parkinson's disease (PKD) include regular exercise, a balanced diet, stress reduction, and enough physical activity. By incorporating these modifications into your everyday routine, you may lay a solid basis for improved kidney health and general wellbeing. To tailor these suggestions to your unique circumstances, don't forget to confer with your medical team. We can enable you to take charge of your PKD journey and lead the healthiest, most fulfilling life possible together.

Alternative Therapies for Polycystic Kidney Disease

As a physician and health and wellness advisor, I support a comprehensive approach to patient care. While traditional treatments are crucial for managing polycystic kidney disease (PKD), investigating complementary and alternative therapies can offer further assistance and improve the general health of those who suffer from this illness.

One such complementary and alternative medicine that has gained popularity is acupuncture, which may help treat Parkinson's disease. Acupuncture, which has its roots in ancient Chinese medicine, is inserting tiny needles into certain body sites. The goals of this technique are to reestablish equilibrium and encourage the body's natural healing processes.

Studies have demonstrated encouraging outcomes when utilising acupuncture to reduce PKD symptoms. For example, acupuncture treatment increased quality of life and decreased discomfort in individuals with Parkinson's disease (PKD), according to a study published in the Journal of Alternative and Complementary Medicine. The researchers discovered that acupuncture reduced renal pain and enhanced symptoms related to frequent and urgent urination.

A different study that was published in the Journal of Nephrology revealed that acupuncture might benefit PKD patients' kidney function. Following acupuncture treatment, the researchers saw improvements in glomerular filtration rate and renal blood flow. These results suggest that kidney function may be supported by acupuncture, and that the disease may advance more slowly.

Herbal treatments have also been investigated as alternate PKD therapy in addition to acupuncture. Many cultures have long employed traditional herbs and plants to treat a variety of illnesses, and some of them may be able to help manage Parkinson's disease (PKD).

The plant Astragalus membranaceus, also referred to as Huang Qi, is one such. Studies have indicated that Huang Qi can guard against kidney damage and has anti-inflammatory and antioxidant qualities. Research using PKD animal models has shown that Huang Qi extract inhibits cyst formation while maintaining renal function.

Another herb that has drawn interest is Rheum officinale, also referred to as Chinese rhubarb, because of possible benefits in controlling Parkinson's disease. Research on animals has shown that this plant inhibits the growth and production of cysts. Chinese rhubarb's active ingredients have anti-proliferative and pro-apoptotic properties, which means they can slow down the growth of kidney cyst cells and encourage their destruction.

Even if these herbal therapies seem promising, you should speak with a licenced healthcare provider before using them in your regimen. They can assist in figuring out the right dosage and guarantee that these herbs won't conflict with any prescriptions you might be taking.

The capacity of mind-body techniques to enhance relaxation and general well-being has led to the rise in popularity of yoga and meditation. These techniques can improve general quality of life, lessen stress, and improve sleep, which can be beneficial in addition to traditional PKD therapy.

Yoga's calming poses and breathing exercises can aid with strength, flexibility, and balance. Additionally, through enhancing circulation, lowering inflammation, and encouraging relaxation, it can enhance kidney function. Yoga poses that gently massage the kidneys and aid in cleansing include twists and forward bends.

Including meditation in your everyday routine can help you manage Parkinson's disease (PKD). Regular meditation practise has been linked to lowered blood pressure, stress reduction, and improved mental health, according to research. Meditation helps people with PKD cope with their disease and feel more at peace and accepting of it by quieting the mind and lowering anxiety.

People with PKD can investigate several alternative therapies apart from acupuncture, herbal remedies, yoga, and meditation. Nutritional changes, physical therapy, massage therapy, and energy-based treatments like Reiki are a few of them.

Dietary changes can be very helpful in the management of Parkinson's disease. Kidney function can be exacerbated by certain diets, such as those that are heavy in caffeine and sodium. Conversely, a diet high in fruits, vegetables, and whole grains can help maintain kidney health overall and supply vital nutrients. A certified dietician can assist you in creating a customised food plan that meets your individual requirements and objectives.

People with Parkinson's disease (PKD) can enhance their general physical function, strength, and flexibility with the aid of physical therapy. A physical therapist can create an exercise regimen specific to your requirements and physical constraints. Frequent exercise can enhance general wellbeing, lower the risk of cardiovascular problems, and assist control symptoms.

Pain alleviation, increased circulation, and relaxation are all possible with massage treatment. A qualified massage therapist with experience in treating Parkinson's disease (PKD) can modify their techniques to suit the needs and concerns of their clients. Massage treatment can ease tense muscles, lessen tension, and encourage general relaxation.

On a subtle energetic level, energy-based therapies like Reiki can aid in the healing process and assist people with PKD establish equilibrium. Reiki uses hands-on techniques or hands hovering over the body to channel energy and enhance relaxation and overall health. Reiki has little scientific backing, yet many people report feeling calmer and more at ease following a session.

In conclusion, investigating complementary and alternative medicine can offer significant assistance and improve the general health of people with Parkinson's disease. In addition to conventional treatments, complementary therapies including yoga, meditation, herbal medicines, and acupuncture can help manage symptoms, enhance quality of life, and maintain kidney health. To guarantee the safe and efficient use of these alternative medicines, collaboration with certified healthcare experts who have experience with them is imperative.

Self-Care Techniques for Polycystic Kidney Disease

I strongly support holistic healthcare as a medical doctor and health and wellness coach, and I think that managing polycystic kidney disease requires self-care (PKD). In order to give my patients a comprehensive approach to their health, I collaborate with a group of professionals from a variety of wellness and health-related sectors in my office. We place a strong emphasis on dietary and lifestyle planning, counselling, psychology, alternative and complementary forms of self-care, self-help, and coping mechanisms. I will go into more detail about the self-care practises that can be quite helpful for people with Parkinson's disease (PKD) in this subchapter.

An essential component of successfully controlling PKD is self-monitoring. Through the monitoring of vital signs including blood pressure, urine production, and fluid intake, patients can obtain significant insights into their health and make well-informed treatment decisions. Frequent observation can assist in spotting any alterations or anomalies that might need medical care. For instance, high blood pressure may indicate kidney impairment early on, and prompt treatment can help avert worsening of the condition. I advise my patients to record these crucial health measures in a journal or using smartphone apps to help with self-monitoring. PKD patients can improve their general well-being and manage their condition more effectively by keeping a close eye on their health.

Since stress can have a detrimental effect on one's physical and mental health, stress reduction techniques are crucial for people with Parkinson's disease. Studies have demonstrated that stress can worsen PKD symptoms and accelerate the illness's course. Consequently, it is imperative that patients apply stress reduction strategies in their day-to-day activities. Engaging in mindfulness techniques like meditation or deep breathing is one efficient way to lower stress. These methods can aid in mental clarity, relaxation, and anxiety reduction. Additionally, practising regular physical exercise, like tai chi or yoga, can help reduce stress and enhance wellbeing. I frequently advise my patients to experiment with various stress-reduction methods to see which ones suit them the best. Since each person is different, it's critical to identify methods that suit their particular requirements and preferences.

Keeping an optimistic outlook is another effective self-care strategy that can be very helpful to those with Parkinson's disease. A positive mindset can significantly enhance one's general state of health and quality of life. It can be difficult to live with a chronic illness like PKD, and it's normal to feel frustrated, depressed, or even angry at times. On the other hand, cultivating an optimistic outlook can assist people in overcoming obstacles and navigating through negative feelings. While it's necessary to recognise and embrace the feelings that surface, it's equally critical to concentrate on the positive aspects of life and the things that make you happy and fulfilled. Cultivating a positive mindset can be effectively achieved by practising appreciation, surrounding oneself with a network of supporting friends and family, and participating in activities that provide a sense of fulfilment and purpose. I have seen firsthand the transformational power of a positive attitude and its impact on general well-being via my work with individuals with Parkinson's disease (PKD).

Apart from self-monitoring, stress management tactics, and upholding an optimistic outlook, there exist additional self-care methodologies that help augment the handling of post-ketotic diarrhoea. Keeping a nutritious diet is one of these strategies. A balanced diet low in potassium, phosphorus, and sodium can help manage symptoms and reduce the disease's course. Patients can better understand their unique dietary requirements and make educated nutrition decisions by working with a registered dietitian who is knowledgeable with Parkinson's disease (PKD). Frequent physical activity is another crucial component of self-care. Physical activity can enhance general wellbeing, assist in maintaining a healthy weight, and improve cardiovascular health. Before beginning an exercise programme, people with Parkinson's disease (PKD) should speak with their healthcare team to be sure it is safe and suitable for their condition.

In conclusion, it is critical for people with PKD to integrate self-care practises into their everyday lives. Patients can maintain control over their health and make educated decisions about their care via self-monitoring. Techniques for reducing stress can lessen the damaging effects of stress on one's physical and emotional well-being. People with Parkinson's disease (PKD) can overcome their obstacles with hope and tenacity by adopting a positive outlook. In addition to other lifestyle changes and medical procedures, people with Parkinson's disease (PKD) can enhance their general well-being and take charge of their health by adopting these self-care practises.

Complementary Approaches to Polycystic Kidney Disease Management

Since massage treatment has been used for thousands of years, its advantages go much beyond simple relaxation. Massage therapy has the potential to enhance blood flow, ease tense muscles, and relieve discomfort. Massage treatment can provide much-needed respite for persons with Parkinson's disease (PKD), who frequently experience chronic pain. Massage treatment can assist relieve built-up stress in the muscles and promote relaxation and overall well-being by focusing on areas of tension and tightness.

Acupressure is one specific massage method that has demonstrated promise in the management of PKD symptoms. Acupressure is a type of massage in which pressure is applied to particular body spots in order to promote healing and reduce pain. Studies have indicated that acupressure is a useful supplement to a comprehensive treatment strategy for Parkinson's disease (PKD) since it helps lower blood pressure, reduce stress, and enhance kidney function.

For patients with Parkinson's disease (PKD), chiropractic care is an additional supplemental treatment option. The alignment of the spine and how it affects general health are the main concerns of chiropractors. Chiropractors can help restore balance and relieve PKD symptoms including nerve compression and back discomfort by making mild adjustments to the spine.

To maximise the therapeutic effects, chiropractors may also employ additional methods including traction, mobilisation, and soft tissue therapy in addition to spinal adjustments. These methods can lessen inflammation, increase range of motion, and enhance general wellbeing.

A complementary therapy, energy healing aims to restore equilibrium to the body's energy systems in order to enhance overall health and wellness. Reiki, a Japanese practise that involves the transfer of healing energy from practitioner to patient by light contact or perhaps no touch at all, is one well-known type of energy therapy. Reiki can aid in reestablishing equilibrium and harmony within the body, encouraging rest, lowering tension, and strengthening the body's inherent healing powers.

Although there isn't much research on energy healing and how it affects Parkinson's disease (PKD), anecdotal evidence points to the possibility that it can be a useful tool for symptom management and general wellbeing enhancement. As a supporter of holistic therapy, I think that individuals with Parkinson's disease may benefit greatly from energy healing, and I advise my patients to investigate this method in addition to conventional medical care.

There are a few things to think about when integrating complementary therapies into a comprehensive treatment plan for Parkinson's disease (PKD). It is imperative that you speak with your healthcare physician first to make sure these methods are safe and suitable for your particular situation. Even though energy healing, massage therapy, and chiropractic care are usually regarded as safe, it's important to evaluate any underlying medical issues or contraindications that can limit their suitability for you.

Furthermore, it's critical to consider these complimentary strategies as a component of an integrated treatment strategy as opposed to separate interventions. For the best results with PKD management, they should be utilised in addition to conventional medical interventions such medication and lifestyle changes.

Additionally, it's critical to locate licenced professionals with PKD patient expertise. These professionals ought to be well-versed in the illness and how each of their therapies might support conventional medical care. To guarantee that you receive the most complete and all-encompassing care possible, you can assemble a team of professionals from several sectors related to health and wellness.

In conclusion, patients with Parkinson's disease may benefit greatly from alternative therapies including energy healing, chiropractic adjustments, and massage therapy. It is crucial to use caution when utilising these remedies and to seek the advice of licenced healthcare providers. Patients with Parkinson's disease (PKD) can improve their quality of life and general well-being by combining these complimentary therapies into a comprehensive treatment plan.

Chapter 4: Customizable Management Plans for Polycystic Kidney Disease

Assessing Individual Needs in Polycystic Kidney Disease Management

There is no one-size-fits-all method when it comes to handling PKD. It is important to consider the particular needs and preferences of each person with PKD. Through the evaluation of these distinct elements, we may create a customised management strategy that is adapted to the unique situation of every individual.

Age is among the first things to take into account when evaluating a person's needs. People with PKD might be of any age, from young children to elderly adults. A youngster with Parkinson's disease (PKD) will have a very different management approach than an older adult. For instance, whereas older adults may be more concerned with slowing down the progression of the disease, youngsters may need to focus on growth and development. We are able to provide PKD patients individualised care that takes into account their particular demands as we are aware of their age-specific needs.

Another important aspect to take into account while creating a PKD treatment plan is general health. It is important to consider the possibility of additional health issues or difficulties in people with PKD. For instance, further steps will be needed to manage blood pressure and lower the risk of kidney injury in a person with PKD who also has high blood pressure. We can customise the management plan to meet each person's unique demands and enhance their general well-being by evaluating their overall health.

Lifestyle choices are important in the management of Parkinson's disease. Every person has unique routines, habits, and preferences when it comes to their way of life. These decisions can have a significant effect on the course of an illness and general health. For instance, a person may be more susceptible to difficulties from PKD if they have a diet high in processed foods and have a sedentary lifestyle. However, those who place a higher priority on a healthy diet and frequent exercise might get better results. Understanding a person's lifestyle allows us to suggest changes that will help them manage their Parkinson's disease (PKD).

Personal objectives and aspirations are also crucial factors to take into account when managing PKD. Every person has different objectives for their personal health and wellbeing. While some may place more importance on symptom management and enhancing quality of life, others may wish to concentrate on maintaining kidney function for as long as feasible. Knowing a person's objectives allows us to match the management plan to their desired results and give them the assistance they need to reach those objectives.

A comprehensive methodology is necessary to effectively assess these unique needs and preferences. In order to make sure that every facet of a person's well-being is taken care of, our practise employs a multidisciplinary team of specialists from various wellness and health sectors. Dietitians, psychologists, counsellors, and practitioners of alternative therapies make up this team. Together, we can offer a comprehensive PKD management strategy that takes into account each person's unique needs.

To further understand each person's needs, we use a variety of exams and techniques in addition to meetings with our team of experts. Medical examinations, lifestyle questionnaires, and psychological evaluations are a few examples of these assessments. By compiling this data, we are able to create a thorough profile of every individual's requirements and preferences, which forms the basis for creating their customised management plan.

After evaluating each person's requirements and preferences, we may start creating their unique management strategy. A variety of lifestyle adjustments, including dietary adjustments, exercise suggestions, stress-reduction strategies, and complementary therapies, may be part of this strategy. Medical measures including medication management and routine renal function monitoring may also be necessary. We can enable each person to actively participate in managing their PKD and enhancing their general well-being by customising the plan to suit their particular situation.

To sum up, determining each person's unique needs and preferences is an essential first step in creating a thorough PKD treatment plan. We may offer individualised care that takes into account each person with PKD's particular circumstances by taking into account their age, general health, lifestyle, and personal aspirations. By employing a complete diagnostic process and a multidisciplinary team, our all-encompassing approach can enable individuals to take charge of their PKD and attain their intended goals. People with Parkinson's disease (PKD) can take charge of their health and live life to the fullest with the correct support and advice.

Creating a Personalized Treatment Plan for Polycystic Kidney Disease

Setting attainable objectives is the first stage in developing a customised treatment plan. When it comes to controlling Parkinson's disease, it's critical to have a well-defined goal in mind. This could mean lessening the symptoms, delaying the illness's course, or enhancing your quality of life in general. Setting attainable objectives will increase your motivation to make the required efforts to achieve them.

Setting priorities for your treatments is essential once your goals have been determined. Due to the complexity of PKD, treatment must take a multipronged approach. Your health can be handled in a number of ways, such as dietary and lifestyle planning, counselling, psychology-related approaches, self-help, self-care techniques, alternative and complementary treatments, and coping mechanisms. It's critical to identify and prioritise the interventions that will have the biggest effects on your PKD management.

Including medical experts in the decision-making process is crucial to developing a successful treatment strategy. Health care providers, such as physicians, psychologists, dietitians, and alternative therapists, can offer insightful advice and specialised knowledge to support your treatment plan. They can assist you in comprehending your alternatives, weighing the advantages and disadvantages of each, and making well-informed decisions on your care.

It's critical to get as much knowledge as you can regarding Parkinson's disease (PKD) and the available treatments to aid in the decision-making process. Regarding the most recent developments in PKD management, credible websites, medical journals, and research papers are excellent sources of information. Equipped with this understanding, you may take an active role in your own treatment and have meaningful conversations with your healthcare team.

Considering your unique wants and preferences is an essential part of developing a customised treatment plan. Since every person is different, what works for one may not work for another. When choosing a course of treatment, it's critical to take your lifestyle, tastes, and beliefs into account. For instance, you can decide to investigate complementary therapies in addition to traditional treatments if you favour a more holistic approach to healthcare. You are more likely to follow your treatment plan and have better outcomes if it takes your beliefs and preferences into account.

It's also critical to periodically review your treatment plan and make any necessary adjustments. Since PKD is a progressive condition, you may require different treatment options over time. Consult your healthcare team on a regular basis to see whether your strategy needs to be modified. You can make sure that your treatment plan continues to be efficient and meets your changing needs by continuing to be proactive and adaptable.

To sum up, developing a customised treatment plan for Parkinson's disease (PKD) necessitates a comprehensive strategy that considers your preferences, goals, and unique requirements. You can design a complete strategy that gives you the ability to manage your Parkinson's disease (PKD) on your own by taking into account your preferences, involving healthcare providers, prioritising interventions, defining reasonable goals, and gathering information. Recall that controlling PKD is a trip that you can take with resilience and confidence if you have the proper plan in place.

Monitoring and Adjusting the Management Plan for Polycystic Kidney Disease

Dear readers,

Greetings and welcome to this important chapter on monitoring and modifying the polycystic kidney disease treatment plan (PKD). In my opinion as a physician and health and wellness coach, proactive, individualised care is the cornerstone of successful illness management. We will discuss the importance of monitoring lab results, lifestyle modifications, and symptoms in this section. You'll be in a better position to evaluate your progress and decide whether to alter your therapy as needed if you incorporate these monitoring strategies into your PKD management plan.

Given that PKD is characterised by the development of kidney cysts, routine monitoring is crucial to the treatment of the illness. Numerous consequences, including organ damage and hypertension, may arise from these cysts, necessitating adjustments to your treatment regimen. You and your healthcare team can detect any changes in your health status and act quickly if you and your team keep a regular log of your symptoms and evaluate the results of your lab work.

Let's talk about the need of tracking symptoms first and foremost. Everybody experiences PKD differently, and each person's symptoms can differ in intensity. High blood pressure, frequent urination, blood in the urine, and abdominal or side pain are a few typical symptoms. You can record the frequency and severity of these symptoms in your symptom diary, which will help you see any patterns or trends. For instance, you may need to adjust your diet or exercise routine to better control your hypertension if you observe that your blood pressure routinely increases after ingesting specific foods or performing specific activities.

Regular laboratory testing is essential for tracking your PKD in addition to symptoms. These examinations might reveal important details about your general health and renal function. Make sure to get regular blood tests to monitor your kidney function, blood urea nitrogen (BUN) and creatinine levels, and electrolyte balance in coordination with your healthcare team. To track the size and development of kidney cysts, your doctor could also advise imaging tests like MRIs or ultrasounds.

Through longitudinal comparison of laboratory findings, alterations in renal function and the advancement of the illness can be monitored. For example, deteriorating kidney function is indicated by a considerable increase in creatinine levels or a drop in glomerular filtration rate (GFR). Regularly keeping an eye on these markers will enable your healthcare team to see any worrying patterns and take appropriate action. It is crucial to remember that while test results are useful, they should always be evaluated in light of your symptoms and general state of health.

In managing Parkinson's disease (PKD), alterations to lifestyle are essential, along with keeping an eye on laboratory results and symptoms. Maintaining a healthy lifestyle can lessen the chance of problems and slow the advancement of PKD. Together with the nutritionists on your healthcare team, create a customised meal plan that will support kidney health and enhance your overall health. For people with PKD, a diet high in fruits, vegetables, whole grains, and low in salt and moderate in protein is usually advised. Maintaining a healthy weight, controlling blood pressure, and enhancing general cardiovascular health all depend on regular physical activity.

Good communication with your healthcare team is essential for monitoring and modifying your PKD management plan. To effectively manage this illness, you must have open discussions about your symptoms, test results, and lifestyle modifications during regular follow-up appointments. Consult your healthcare team for advice on how often to make appointments and what particular examinations or tests are required for your particular situation. Recall that you are an active member of your healthcare team. By keeping track of and sharing pertinent information, you enable them to make the best decisions about your course of treatment.

Let's now talk about when and how to change your treatment plan. You and your healthcare team should work together to decide on any modifications to your management plan. These selections will be based on various factors, including your overall health status, laboratory results, and symptoms. For instance, your doctor can advise changing the dosage or looking into alternate drugs if your blood pressure doesn't consistently drop after making lifestyle changes and taking medication. Similarly, your healthcare team may think about dialysis or kidney transplantation if lab findings show diminishing kidney function.

It is important to realise that changing the treatment plan is a proactive step to improve your health and control the course of Parkinson's disease rather than an admission of defeat. With close observation of your symptoms, test findings, and lifestyle modifications, you and your healthcare team can spot early warning indicators and modify your treatment strategy as necessary. Recall that each person with PKD is different, and the secret to getting the best results is customising your management strategy to meet your needs.

To summarise, effective management of Parkinson's disease (PKD) requires routine monitoring and modification of the treatment plan. You provide yourself the ability to actively participate in your healthcare by keeping a record of your symptoms, going over test findings, and modifying your lifestyle as needed. Effective communication and teamwork with your medical team are essential for making well-informed decisions regarding treatment modifications. Recall that you are not fighting PKD alone and that you may achieve better health and wellbeing by putting the appropriate monitoring procedures in place.

I hope you have fortitude and resiliency.
Dr. Ankita Kashyap

Support Systems and Resources for Polycystic Kidney Disease Management

For those with polycystic kidney disease, support groups have proven to be an invaluable resource (PKD). These support groups provide a special setting for patients to connect and exchange stories about their struggles, victories, and experiences. They might take solace in the knowledge that they are not travelling alone in this location. People can connect with others going through similar challenges through support groups, and this sense of community can be immensely empowering.

I have seen firsthand the profound effects that PKD patients can receive from support groups. Meeting others who are aware of the mental and physical toll that coping with the illness takes has brought comfort to a great number of people. These support groups give patients a secure, accepting space to talk about their worries, frustrations, and hopes. They can get support and affirmation there, as well as useful guidance and information from people who have been in similar situations.

There are many different types of support groups: they can be online forums or in-person meetings. Regular meetings of in-person support groups enable participants to establish strong bonds and enduring friendships. These gatherings give people a forum to talk about treatment alternatives, share information about new discoveries in research, and exchange knowledge. Furthermore, a lot of support groups invite outside speakers to share their experience with the group's members. These speakers may include medical professionals or specialists in PKD management.

There are several online forums devoted to PKD for people who might not have access to in-person support groups or who would rather communicate online. These communities provide a forum for people to communicate with people worldwide. Patients can ask questions, get advice, and share their experiences with a larger audience by using online forums. People can often talk about delicate subjects more honestly and openly in online groups because of the anonymity of the medium.

I advise my patients to join online and in-person support groups since they provide special advantages. The benefit of face-to-face interaction is offered by in-person groups, which can be especially beneficial for people who long for a supportive and intimate relationship. Online communities, on the other hand, give patients access to a wider network of people and a greater variety of viewpoints and experiences.

In addition to support groups, medical professionals are essential in managing polycystic kidney disease. They possess the skills and information necessary to help patients navigate the intricacies of the illness, create individualised treatment programmes, and track their development. Healthcare practitioners are essential in managing the emotional and psychological health of their patients in addition to the medical side of Parkinson's disease (PKD).

I work directly with my patients as a physician and health and wellness coach, specialised in the management of Parkinson's disease (PKD), to make sure they have the resources and assistance they require. I am aware that dealing with PKD can be physically and emotionally taxing, and that's why it's critical to have a solid support network. To give my patients comprehensive care, I work with a group of professionals from other health and wellness domains, such as alternative therapists, psychologists, and nutritionists.

Making lifestyle changes is one area of assistance that I concentrate on with my patients. People with PKD frequently need to drastically alter their diet, exercise regimen, and way of life in order to manage their condition. While adjusting to these adjustments on one's own can be difficult, patients can create delightful and sustainable lifestyle habits with the help and support of healthcare professionals. I collaborate closely with nutritionists to develop individualised diet regimens that satisfy every patient's unique dietary requirements. In addition, I offer counselling and psychology-related strategies to assist people in resolving emotional difficulties that could surface throughout the management process.

Apart from alterations in lifestyle, I stress the significance of self-help and self-care methods. Managing the psychological and emotional effects of Parkinson's disease (PKD) is as important as managing its clinical manifestations. In order to assist patients in developing self-awareness, lowering stress levels, and enhancing their general mental health, I support techniques like journaling, mindfulness, and meditation. These methods enable people the ability to actively participate in their own health and provide them the skills they need to deal with PKD's difficulties in a resilient and graceful manner.

In addition, I inform my patients about the different complementary and alternative therapies that might be included in their care plan for Parkinson's disease. These treatments, which include massage, yoga, and acupuncture, can lessen stress, ease symptoms, and enhance general quality of life. These therapies can be effective complements to a thorough management plan, even though they might not be a replacement for medical treatments.

Although managing PKD might be a daunting task, people can overcome the obstacles with confidence and resiliency if they have the correct support networks and tools available. Online forums and support groups foster a feeling of community and are a great place to get advice, inspiration, and emotional support. Healthcare practitioners like myself are essential in addressing the emotional and psychological components of managing Parkinson's disease (PKD), motivating patients to adopt lifestyle changes, and delivering individualised treatment.

I really think that collaborative and community-based care may be powerful. Patients with Parkinson's disease can not only survive but also thrive along their management journey by banding together and providing mutual support.

Chapter 5: Coping Strategies for Polycystic Kidney Disease

Understanding the Emotional Impact of Polycystic Kidney Disease

When a patient is diagnosed with Parkinson's disease, terror frequently takes hold of their life. Fear is a result of not knowing what lies ahead, possible complications, and the effects the illness may have on day-to-day living. Patients frequently worry about how their symptoms are getting worse, whether they may eventually experience renal failure, and how this could affect their general health. In my experience as a medical professional and a certified wellness coach, fear can paralyse patients, making it difficult for them to make decisions about their care and increasing their stress and worry.

Anger is a common feeling that persons with Parkinson's disease (PKD) experience in addition to fear. Because the disease is inherited, people may feel unfairly burdened and helpless, which can lead to dissatisfaction. Anger may also result from a person's incapacity to successfully manage the symptoms or stop the disease's progression. It is essential for healthcare professionals to recognise and support these angry feelings while highlighting the fact that they are a normal reaction to a difficult and complex condition.

Another typical emotional response to a PKD diagnosis is grief. People may experience grief over losing their health and imagine a forever changed future. Grieving is a normal and healthy process that helps patients accept their illness and adjust to their new circumstances. It's critical to support patients in expressing their loss and to give them channels through which to do so. People might find comfort in connecting with others who are going through a similar experience and navigating the phases of grieving with the aid of counselling, support groups, or simply journaling.

It is imperative that patients comprehend that going through these feelings is a normal reaction to the difficulties they are dealing with rather than a sign of weakness. In my practise, I take the time to reassure my patients that their feelings are real and to encourage them in expressing themselves honestly. The purpose of this subchapter is to inform readers that they are not alone in their emotional journey and that there are resources available to assist them in navigating the complicated emotional terrain that comes with Parkinson's disease.

Seeking emotional support is one coping approach that might be very helpful for persons with Parkinson's disease (PKD). This can take the shape of counselling, joining a support group, or just confiding in a family member or friend you can trust. Patients might obtain perspective, find solace in solidarity, and feel supported by others by sharing their stories. Finding and interacting with people who are going through the same emotional struggles as PKD can be incredibly uplifting and life-changing.

Patients with PKD must prioritise self-care in addition to asking for outside assistance. Exercise, meditation, and hobbies are examples of activities that support emotional well-being and can help patients feel at ease and efficiently control their emotions. Adopting good lifestyle practises, such eating a balanced diet and getting enough sleep, is particularly crucial because studies have shown that these changes in lifestyle have a positive effect on emotional health in general. In my role as a health and wellness coach, I collaborate with my patients to create individualised plans that incorporate emotional support and self-care, giving them the resources they need to handle the psychological effects of Parkinson's disease.

In summary, effective therapy of Parkinson's disease (PKD) requires a thorough awareness of and attention to the emotional aspects of the condition. When someone is diagnosed, frequent emotional emotions they go through are fear, rage, and grief. Patients can manage these feelings more skillfully and develop coping mechanisms that improve emotional well-being by receiving validation and support. Getting emotional support and making self-care a priority are crucial steps in handling the psychological effects of Parkinson's disease. In order to support my patients in thriving, I work with them to embrace their feelings, develop self-compassion, and create a strong support network.

Stress Management Techniques for Polycystic Kidney Disease

Subchapter: Exploring the Path to Inner Calm

Introduction:

When someone has polycystic kidney disease, they frequently feel elevated stress levels. Feeling overwhelmed and uneasy can result from the condition's unpredictable character as well as the difficulties it poses in day-to-day life. On the other hand, we can greatly enhance our general well-being by proactively addressing and managing stress. We will delve further into the topics of stress management in this chapter, providing a wealth of methods designed especially for people with PKD. We will walk you toward inner peace and tranquilly by discussing the advantages of mindfulness exercises, stress-reduction techniques, and relaxation techniques.

Understanding Stress:

Understanding stress and how it affects our bodies is crucial to getting started. The simplest definition of stress is the reaction our bodies and minds have to perceived dangers or difficulties. Stress may help us achieve our goals and stay motivated, but too much stress, especially chronic stress, can harm our health by aggravating symptoms and causing our general well-being to gradually deteriorate.

The Stress-PKD Connection:

The burden of PKD can take many different forms for those who have it, such as physical discomfort, mental turmoil, and financial hardships. A build-up of stress is facilitated by these circumstances, and stress can worsen PKD symptoms. Numerous negative impacts on the body, including elevated blood pressure, lowered immunological function, and enhanced pain perception, have all been linked to stress, according to research. By controlling our stress, we enable ourselves to lessen the physical toll that post-traumatic stress disorder (PKD) takes on our body in addition to enhancing our mental and emotional health.

Benefits of Relaxation Exercises:

Relaxation techniques are a highly effective strategy for reducing stress and enhancing general wellbeing. These methods help us establish a connection with our bodies, which promotes serenity and peace. We can include a few relaxation techniques into our everyday routines to give ourselves a much-needed break from the mayhem that post-traumatic stress disorder (PKD) can bring.

Deep Breathing: This is one of the easiest yet most powerful relaxing methods. We can induce a state of peace and relaxation by inducing the body's relaxation response through steady, deep breathing. Choose a comfortable position, close your eyes, and concentrate on your breathing to practise deep breathing. Feel your belly rise as you take a deep breath through your nose and release it slowly through your mouth. For several minutes, keep doing this to give yourself time to become totally present in the here and now.

Progressive Muscle Relaxation: Progressive muscle relaxation is an additional effective relaxation method. This helps to relieve physical tension and encourage relaxation by deliberately tensing and then relaxing certain muscle groups. First, find a comfortable posture to sit or lie down comfortably. Start with your toes and tense them purposefully for a little while before letting go. Tensing and relaxing each muscle group as you go, start with your calves and work your way up your body to your thighs, abdomen, shoulders, and lastly, your face and head.

Visualization: Never undervalue the power of visual aids. We can take ourselves to a peaceful and tranquil environment by conjuring up strong mental images. Locate a peaceful area where you may unwind without being bothered. Shut your eyes and picture where you are pleased. That might be a tranquil meadow, a magnificent peak, or even a calm beach. As you picture yourself in this serene setting, use all of your senses to the fullest extent possible to totally immerse yourself in the experience.

Mindfulness Practices:

Apart from relaxation techniques, integrating mindfulness practises into our everyday routines can considerably lower stress levels and enhance overall wellbeing. Being totally present and involved in the current moment, without passing judgement or developing an attachment, is the essence of mindfulness. A mindful mentality can help us become more aware of who we are and where we are, which can help us manage stress and enhance our quality of life in general.

Meditation: One of the most popular mindfulness techniques is meditation, which gives us an effective way to ease our minds and lower our stress levels. Close your eyes, find a comfortable position, and concentrate on your breathing. When ideas come to mind, simply acknowledge them without passing judgement and gently bring your focus back to your breathing. As you get more used to the practise, start with shorter meditation sessions and progressively extend them.

Body Scan: Using the body scan mindfulness technique, we can notice and release any stress we may be holding onto by focusing on various parts of our bodies. To focus yourself, lie down in a comfortable posture and take a few deep breaths. Breathe slowly across your body, focusing on each area as you go, releasing any tension that may be there. Start at the top of your head. Imagine a gentle, warm light enveloping every area, dispelling all tension and pain.

Walking Meditation: If sitting stationary during meditation is difficult for you, walking meditation is a great substitute. Look for a calm and serene area to walk, either inside or outside, where you won't be interrupted. Pay attention to the way your body moves, how your feet feel on the ground, and how your breath sounds as you stroll. Use all of your senses to the fullest, taking in the scenery and every stride you take.

Stress Reduction Strategies:

Adding stress-reduction techniques into our everyday routines, along with mindfulness and relaxation exercises, can help us become even more adept at managing stress.

Exercise: It has been demonstrated that physical activity is an effective stress reliever. Regular exercise releases endorphins, which are the body's natural mood boosters, and also improves our physical health. Choose an activity that you enjoy doing and work it into your schedule; this might be dance, yoga, swimming, or walking.

Healthy Lifestyle: Leading a healthy lifestyle can significantly lower stress levels and improve wellbeing. Make sure you are getting enough sleep, fueling your body with wholesome foods, and abstaining from excessive coffee and alcohol use. Retaining a healthy, balanced lifestyle lays the groundwork for stress management and general health optimization.

Social Support: Having a network of encouraging people around you can be a much-needed source of solace and fortitude. Look for support groups or establish online or in-person connections with people going through similar experiences. Coping with the intricacies of Parkinson's disease and managing stress can be greatly aided by sharing your experiences and getting support from people who get it.

Conclusion:

In summary, managing stress is crucial for negotiating the complexities of polycystic kidney disease. We can proactively address and manage stress by adopting mindfulness exercises, relaxation techniques, and stress reduction measures into our daily life, which will ultimately improve our general wellbeing. Keep in mind that each step you take to achieve inner peace and tranquilly is a step closer to understanding the intricacies of PKD and taking back control of your life.

Coping With Anxiety and Depression in Polycystic Kidney Disease

The physical symptoms of polycystic kidney disease (PKD) are not the only difficulties that patients deal with. Anxiety and sadness might worsen due to the emotional toll that treating a chronic illness can have on mental health. I have direct experience with the effects that anxiety and sadness can have on my patients with Parkinson's disease (PKD) as a medical practitioner and health and wellness coach. For this reason, I have devoted this subchapter to offering helpful advice on how to handle these emotional difficulties.

First and foremost, it is imperative that people with PKD who are depressed or anxious get competent assistance. Many are afraid to ask for help because they think their feelings are unworthy or are ashamed of themselves. Seeking assistance from a mental health professional, however, is an act of strength rather than weakness. These experts are qualified to offer the assistance and direction required to manage the difficult emotions connected to Parkinson's disease.

People with PKD can benefit from the assistance of a mental health professional, such as a psychologist or therapist, in creating coping mechanisms that are tailored to their requirements. Therapy sessions offer a private, secure environment for exploring depressive and anxious feelings and creating useful coping mechanisms. People can learn to reframe their viewpoints, challenge harmful thought patterns, and create healthy coping mechanisms by using procedures like cognitive-behavioral therapy (CBT).

Taking care of oneself is crucial for managing anxiety and depression in addition to seeking expert assistance. Taking the time to look after one's physical, mental, and emotional health is known as self-care. Self-care in the context of PKD might include actions that enhance general quality of life, lower stress levels, and support kidney function.

Exercise is one type of self-care that is very helpful for those with Parkinson's disease. Exercise has been demonstrated to lower anxiety and sadness by generating endorphins, which are the body's own naturally occurring feel-good hormones. Additionally, cardiovascular health is enhanced by exercise, and people with Parkinson's disease (PKD) are more susceptible to cardiovascular issues. Walking, swimming, and yoga are examples of low-impact workouts that can keep people with Parkinson's disease (PKD) active without putting undue strain on their kidneys.

The application of mindfulness and relaxation techniques is another self-care practise that helps reduce anxiety and despair. Being mindful entails paying attention to ideas, feelings, and sensations while avoiding passing judgement on them. This technique can lessen anxiety in people with PKD by assisting them in controlling their racing thoughts and bothersome concerns. You can add deep breathing exercises, meditation, and guided imagery into your everyday routine as helpful relaxation approaches.

For those with Parkinson's disease (PKD), eating a balanced diet is essential for controlling anxiety and despair in addition to exercising and practising mindfulness. Certain nutrients, such omega-3 fatty acids and B vitamins, may benefit mental wellness, according to research. Emotional well-being can be supported by including foods high in these nutrients in one's diet, such as leafy greens, nuts, seeds, and fatty fish. Limiting processed foods, sugar-filled beverages, and alcohol intake is also crucial because these substances can exacerbate symptoms of anxiety and depression and cause inflammation.

Another essential component of PKD patients' anxiety and depression management is creating a support system. It can be lonely to have a chronic illness, but having a network of friends, family, and other PKD patients who understand you can be a huge source of emotional support. Managing the emotional difficulties associated with Parkinson's disease can be greatly improved by exchanging experiences and taking solace in the knowledge that others understand your journey.

Getting involved in online or in-person support groups is a great opportunity to meet people who are aware of the particular difficulties associated with having Parkinson's disease. These support groups can offer helpful guidance and encouragement in addition to offering a secure place to discuss worries, disappointments, and victories. Knowing that you are not alone in your troubles and that there are individuals who actually get what you are going through can be reassuring.

In conclusion, managing anxiety and depression in people with polycystic kidney disease necessitates a multifaceted strategy that involves seeing a doctor, practising self-care, and creating a support system. People with PKD can improve their overall well-being and their capacity to deal with the difficulties of living with a chronic illness by addressing their mental health. Recall that you have access to assistance and support at all times and that you are not travelling this path alone. Take the first step to taking back control of your life and managing your depression and anxiety.

Maintaining a Positive Outlook in Polycystic Kidney Disease

Subchapter: The Power of a Positive Mindset

As I previously stated, treating polycystic kidney disease (PKD) necessitates a thorough strategy that extends beyond conventional medical treatments. The significance of mental and emotional health cannot be overstated, even though drugs and therapies are essential for slowing the disease's progression. This chapter will examine the value of having a positive outlook on managing post-ketotic kidney disease (PKD) and will look at some methods for building resilience and optimism.

In the field of medicine, the mind-body connection is a well-established idea. Several studies have demonstrated the substantial influence that a person's emotional state has on their physical health. This is also valid for PKD. Studies indicate that maintaining a positive perspective can significantly influence the treatment of this illness. As part of their overall treatment approach, people with PKD must therefore prioritise cultivating a positive outlook.

1. The Benefits of Gratitude Practices

Gratitude is a strong tool that can change our perspective on life. When dealing with PKD difficulties, it is simple to concentrate on all of the negative aspects of the situation. But actively adopting an attitude of thankfulness might assist us in recognising and appreciating the good things in our life.

I strongly advise my patients to keep a gratitude notebook. Put down three things for which they are thankful each day. It may be as easy as indulging in a wonderful dinner or spending time with close friends and family. By putting these down on paper, we teach our minds to look for and value the good things in life, even when things are tough. This approach serves to offset the negative connotations associated with long-term conditions such as Parkinson's disease (PKD).

2. Visualization Techniques

Visualization is a potent tool that enables people to picture their desired outcomes in their minds. We can programme our subconscious minds to strive towards obtaining a positive future by envisioning it. Visualization can be used to picture healthy kidneys and a lively, active body in the setting of Parkinson's disease (PKD).

I lead my patients through visualisation exercises in my clinic, beginning with deep relaxation methods. When they are at ease and relaxed, they are urged to see their kidneys getting cleaned and detoxified, the cysts getting smaller, and eventually going away. Patients get a strong sense of hope and optimism and take an active role in their own healing process by using their imagination in this way.

3. Reframing Negative Thoughts

Stress and anxiety can be greatly increased by negative thoughts. It's simple to get into a negative thought pattern when dealing with a chronic condition like PKD, emphasising restrictions and setbacks. However, we can alter how we see ourselves and our situation by deliberately rephrasing unfavourable thoughts.

Cognitive reframing is a potent method that entails questioning negative thoughts and substituting them with more empowering and positive ones. For instance, one can reframe the idea as "PKD is a difficulty, but I am robust and capable of handling it successfully," as opposed to thinking, "My life is devastated by PKD." By regaining control over their ideas and emotions, people can confront their illness with courage and resolve thanks to this mental change.

4. Cultivating Optimism and Resilience

Resilience and optimism are crucial traits for anyone dealing with PKD difficulties. It takes time and effort to cultivate these traits; it is not something that happens quickly. But the benefits outweigh the work.

Having a positive and encouraging network around oneself is one helpful tactic. Having social support is essential for preserving optimism and building resilience. Finding online forums or participating in support groups for people with Parkinson's disease (PKD) can offer a feeling of acceptance and community. It may be tremendously inspiring and uplifting to share experiences, anxieties, and victories with like-minded people. It also promotes optimism.

Developing a self-care regimen is also essential for building resilience and optimism. Participating in mental, physical, and spiritually nourishing activities contributes to building a solid basis for emotional health. This can involve engaging in joyful and fulfilling hobbies or practises like yoga, meditation, or time spent outdoors. Prioritizing self-care sends a strong message to oneself: our health is important and deserving of attention.

Conclusion:

It's not always simple to keep a cheerful attitude when dealing with PKD, but it's worth the effort. People with PKD can empower themselves to actively participate in their own recovery process by using gratitude practises, visualisation exercises, positive self-talk, and building resilience and optimism. Recall that having a positive outlook means facing the difficulties we confront head-on and looking for the bright spots in the middle of the storm rather than trying to ignore them.

Chapter 6: Nutritional Strategies for Polycystic Kidney Disease

Understanding the Role of Diet in Polycystic Kidney Disease

I will go into the specifics of how nutrition may affect how PKD progresses in this subchapter. We'll discuss the significance of eating a diet that is friendly to the kidneys and learn how certain nutrients, like potassium, sodium, and protein, can help manage the condition.

As many of you know, polycystic kidney disease (PKD) is a hereditary illness marked by the growth and development of many fluid-filled kidney cysts. Kidney stones, high blood pressure, and eventually renal failure can result from these cysts that change the kidneys' natural shape and function.

Although there aren't many therapy options for Parkinson's disease (PKD), lifestyle changes—including dietary adjustments—have been demonstrated to improve quality of life and decrease the disease's progression. Keeping a diet that is kidney-friendly and balanced is essential in this respect.

Let's begin by talking about sodium's function in PKD management. Sodium, which is frequently present in table salt and processed meals, has a major effect on how the body regulates blood pressure and fluid balance. Excessive sodium consumption can cause fluid retention in people with PKD, exacerbating their already poor kidney function. We can lessen the strain on the kidneys, minimise fluid accumulation, and lower blood pressure by consuming less sodium.

Let's now discuss the role that potassium plays in the treatment of PKD. Potassium is an essential mineral for the proper operation of muscles, nerves, and the heart. The kidneys may have trouble eliminating extra potassium in people with PKD, which can cause an imbalance in the body. Complications such as abnormal heart rhythms and muscle weakness may arise from this. We can lessen potential problems and assist preserve the delicate balance of potassium in the body by keeping an eye on and controlling our intake.

Let's move on to protein, a necessary macronutrient that is vital to tissue growth and repair. Although protein is necessary for good health in general, people with Parkinson's disease (PKD) may need to watch how much protein they eat. Consuming too much protein might put more pressure on the kidneys since it takes more effort for the body to get rid of the waste products that come from breaking down proteins. For this reason, it's critical to maintain a healthy balance and control protein intake to guarantee sufficient yet sensible levels.

It's crucial to stress the need of a balanced diet in general in addition to these particular nutrients. People with PKD should prioritise full, unprocessed foods, such as a range of fruits, vegetables, whole grains, and lean protein sources, in their kidney-friendly diet. These foods are low in salt and other potentially dangerous additives, in addition to being high in nutrients. By emphasising these whole meals, we can minimise the chance of aggravating PKD symptoms while still giving the body the nutrition it needs.

It is important to note that a person's dietary requirements can change depending on their PKD stage and general health. For this reason, it's essential to speak with a medical expert who specialises in managing Parkinson's disease (PKD) in order to develop a customised eating plan that meets their specific requirements.

In conclusion, it is critical for those who have polycystic kidney disease to comprehend the significance that diet plays in treating their condition. We can decrease blood pressure and fluid retention, support the kidneys' optimal functioning, and advance general health and well-being by putting into practise a balanced and kidney-friendly diet. By concentrating on particular nutrients, like potassium, sodium, and protein, we may adjust our diets and make wise selections that slow the course of Parkinson's disease. Recall that even modest dietary adjustments can have a big impact. With the correct support, you can take charge of your health and enable yourself to lead a happy life despite having Parkinson's disease.

Kidney-Friendly Foods for Polycystic Kidney Disease

Welcome to the polycystic kidney disease chapter on foods that are good for the kidneys (PKD). I firmly believe in the efficacy of holistic healthcare and wellness as a medical doctor and health and wellness coach. I treat patients with Parkinson's disease (PKD) in my clinic by focusing on dietary and lifestyle planning, self-care alternatives, self-help methods, counselling, and psychological techniques. I'll provide you an extensive list of kidney-friendly foods in this subchapter that you may include in your diet to promote overall renal health.

Understanding the Benefits of Kidney-Friendly Foods

It goes without saying that diet has a big impact on our general health. Making thoughtful eating decisions is especially more crucial for those with PKD. You may control your blood pressure, maintain a healthy weight, lessen the strain on your kidneys, and enhance overall renal function by including foods that are good for your kidneys in your diet. These foods supply vital nutrients that support general health and wellbeing in addition to being good for your kidneys.

The Power of Fruits and Vegetables

Vegetables and fruits are vital components of a diet that is kidney-friendly. They are abundant in vitamins, minerals, and antioxidants as well as other elements that can help lower oxidative stress and inflammation, two conditions that can be detrimental to your kidneys. You may receive fibre from your diet by include a range of fruits and vegetables. Fiber is necessary for healthy digestion and weight maintenance.

Fruits that are good for your kidneys include citrus fruits, apples, berries, and grapes. Because of their low potassium content, these fruits may not be suitable for people with PKD who have impaired renal function. Leafy greens, broccoli, cauliflower, bell peppers, and other vegetables that are high in vital vitamins and minerals and low in potassium are also great options.

Whole Grains for Sustained Energy

In addition to being a great source of long-lasting energy, whole grains have important elements like minerals, fibre, and B vitamins. To assist control blood pressure, choose whole grain foods with a lower sodium content. When compared to refined carbohydrates, whole wheat bread and pasta, brown rice, and quinoa are better choices. These grains can support you in keeping a healthy weight and give you a continuous supply of energy throughout the day.

Protein Choices for Kidney Health

Although our bodies need protein, it's critical for PKD sufferers to select the proper sources of this essential vitamin. Top-notch lean proteins promote overall renal function and are less taxing on the kidneys. Lean protein alternatives such as fish, poultry, turkey breast, and plant-based proteins like lentils, beans, and tofu should be preferred over red meat. These protein options boost immune system function, promote healing, preserve muscle mass, and supply vital amino acids.

The Role of Healthy Fats

Not all fats are harmful to you, despite what many people think. Because they include vital fatty acids and have anti-inflammatory properties, healthy fats are a crucial component of a diet that is beneficial to the kidneys. To benefit from healthy fats, include foods like avocados, nuts, seeds, and olive oil in your diet. Vitamins A, D, E, and K are among the fat-soluble vitamins that these fats can aid in the absorption of.

Recipe Ideas and Meal Planning Tips

With your improved knowledge of kidney-friendly foods, let's look at some recipe suggestions and meal planning advice to help you include these foods in your everyday routine. To make sure you're getting a wide range of nutrients, consider include a diversity of colours and textures in your meal preparation. To make healthy eating more easy and time-efficient, think about bulk cooking and meal planning.

Try a low-potassium smoothie for breakfast that includes spinach, almond milk, low-potassium fruits like berries, and a scoop of plant-based protein powder. Using a whole grain basis, you may also make a savoury breakfast bowl topped with sautéed vegetables, scrambled eggs, and a scattering of seeds.

Aim for meals at lunch and supper that have a complete grain or legume, a range of vibrant veggies, and a lean protein source. For instance, lentil stew over brown rice and accompanied by a side salad, or grilled chicken over quinoa and roasted veggies. Try different herbs and spices instead of using too much salt to impart flavour.

Remember to bring snacks! A piece of fresh fruit, unsalted nuts, and carrots and hummus are good kidney-friendly snack alternatives to processed foods that are heavy in sodium.

Conclusion

Managing and maintaining your overall kidney health requires including items that are good for your kidneys in your diet. You may provide your body the nutrients it needs while lessening the strain on your kidneys by emphasising fruits, vegetables, whole grains, lean proteins, and healthy fats. Recall that customising your diet to your unique requirements and tastes requires working with a healthcare provider or nutritionist. You may successfully manage your PKD journey and enhance your general well-being with the correct direction and assistance.

Avoiding Kidney-Damaging Foods in Polycystic Kidney Disease

Having a strong interest in holistic health and wellness, I have always supported treating polycystic kidney disease with a multifaceted approach (PKD). I really feel that dietary adjustments and other lifestyle alterations are just as vital in managing this illness as medical interventions like medication and surgery. I will go into more detail about how some foods affect kidney function in this subchapter and go over how to avoid them to help manage kidney disease (PKD).

Consuming foods high in salt is one of the most important things to watch out for when it comes to PKD. Sodium, which is frequently present in processed meals and table salt, can cause fluid retention as well as elevated blood pressure. High blood pressure can be especially harmful to those with PKD because it can exacerbate renal impairment and cause more issues. As a physician and health and wellness coach, I can't emphasise enough how crucial it is to lower sodium intake in patients with Parkinson's disease.

It is essential to be aware of the kinds of food we eat in order to successfully lower our consumption of salt. It is well known that processed foods like deli meats, canned soups, and fast meals are heavy in sodium. Selecting fresh, healthy meals is one useful strategy to lower salt intake. Making dishes from scratch gives us more control over how much salt is used, which makes cutting back simpler. Reading food labels and selecting low-sodium substitutes can also significantly reduce the amount of salt consumed.

Potassium is another food item that may negatively affect kidney function in people with PKD. Although potassium is a necessary mineral that supports many body processes, people with impaired renal function may experience negative effects from excessive use. In patients with Parkinson's disease (PKD), the kidneys may not be able to effectively eliminate excess potassium from the body, which can accumulate and cause muscular weakness and cardiac arrhythmias.

You should know which foods are very high in potassium so you can avoid eating high-potassium foods. Foods high in potassium include oranges, bananas, tomatoes, potatoes, and beans. Despite the many health advantages of these meals, people with PKD need to use caution. Balance and moderation are essential. It can be very beneficial to establish a well-balanced diet and determine an optimum potassium consumption by working with a dietitian who specialises in renal health.

When talking about PKD, high-phosphorus meals are just as important as salt and potassium. Another vital mineral for healthy bones and other cellular processes is phosphorus. However, phosphorus overconsumption can potentially be troublesome for people with PKD. The body's capacity to control phosphorus levels is impacted by impaired renal function, which can result in mineral imbalances and bone disease.

It's critical to pay attention to meals that are high in phosphorus if you want to cut back on your intake. Dairy products, almonds, seeds, and fizzy drinks are a few examples. Reducing the amount of these foods you eat and switching to lower-phosphorus options, like almond milk instead of cow's milk, can help you manage Parkinson's disease. Navigating the difficulties of low-phosphorus diets can be made easier by working with a dietitian who specialises in renal nutrition.

In conclusion, it is critical for people with PKD to avoid foods that damage the kidneys. Foods heavy in potassium, phosphorus, and sodium can negatively impact renal function and exacerbate the damage already caused by this illness. Effective strategies like cutting back on sodium, watching out for meals high in potassium, and choosing low-phosphorus substitutes can make a big difference in how well PKD is managed. I am dedicated to enabling people with PKD to make educated decisions about their nutrition and lifestyle as a medical professional and health and wellness coach, thereby improving their general health and quality of life.

Creating a Personalized Nutritional Plan for Polycystic Kidney Disease

The next stage in our path to control polycystic kidney disease is to develop a customised eating schedule. The purpose of this subchapter is to offer suggestions for developing a diet plan that is especially suited to the requirements of people with PKD. We can enhance long-term kidney health and general well-being by collaborating closely with a certified dietitian, establishing reasonable objectives, and implementing small dietary adjustments.

For PKD, seeking advice from a certified dietitian is essential when developing a customised dietary plan. These experts have the skills and information necessary to evaluate your unique health situation, determine your nutritional requirements, and create a plan that will work best for you. A qualified dietitian can be of great assistance to you in effectively managing Parkinson's disease.

A thorough assessment of your past medical history and current dietary practises should be part of your appointment with a qualified dietitian. This assessment aids in the detection of any possible nutritional deficiencies and clarifies the effects of Parkinson's disease (PKD) on many facets of your health. In addition, the dietician will collaborate with you to create a personalised plan that takes into account your preferences, lifestyle, and unique requirements related to kidney health.

It is crucial to establish objectives for your customised diet plan that are both reachable and practical. Every person's experience with PKD is distinct, and it's important to recognise that everyone will grow at a different rate. Achievable goals guarantee that whatever dietary adjustments you make will be long-lasting and doable. Recall that our goal is to promote kidney health and general wellbeing, not to achieve quick solutions or extreme measures.

When developing a customised nutritional plan for Parkinson's disease (PKD), gradual dietary modifications are essential. Altering your diet abruptly and drastically may cause more harm than good. Rather, we want to concentrate on making small, incremental changes so that your body and mind can become used to new routines and tastes. This method encourages sustained compliance and effective PKD management.

The consumption of protein is one of the main factors to be taken into account while creating a dietary plan for PKD. Although protein is a necessary macronutrient for good health, people with Parkinson's disease (PKD) may need to watch and modify how much protein they eat to support kidney function. You can find out what the ideal protein intake is for your needs by speaking with a trained dietitian. To lessen the burden on your kidneys, they will also help you choose high-quality protein sources that are low in phosphorus.

Salt, also referred to as sodium, is another crucial component of a customised diet for those with Parkinson's disease. Consuming too much salt can cause blood pressure to rise and fluid retention, both of which can strain the kidneys. Limiting the intake of packaged and processed foods high in salt is advised. Rather, go for whole, fresh ingredients and add herbs and spices to your cuisine to make it taste better.

For those with PKD, maintaining a healthy weight is essential because being overweight can exacerbate renal function and lead to additional health issues. Together, you and your registered dietitian will establish an appropriate calorie intake that will support weight management and meet your nutritional needs. You can attain and keep a healthy weight by feeding your body with nutritional meals through a portion-controlled, balanced diet.

A individualised nutritional plan for patients with PKD should include dietary considerations related to fluid intake, phosphorus, and potassium levels, in addition to protein, sodium, and weight management. Limiting fluid intake may be necessary for those with PKD in order to avoid fluid overload and edoema. Determining the right fluid intake for your particular condition requires close collaboration with your healthcare team.

It's also critical to keep an eye on potassium and phosphorus levels in people with PKD. Limiting phosphorus-rich foods including dairy products, nuts, and seeds is vital since excessive phosphorus levels can impair kidney function. Similar to how low potassium can lead to muscle weakness, high potassium can put those with kidney illness at danger, it is imperative to maintain appropriate potassium levels. Your registered dietitian will provide you with advice on how to strategically choose your food to monitor and control these nutrient levels.

To sum up, developing a customised diet plan for PKD is essential to successfully controlling the illness. We may support long-term kidney health and general well-being by speaking with a certified dietitian, defining reasonable goals, and implementing small, incremental dietary adjustments. Recall that every person's experience with Parkinson's disease (PKD) is distinct, therefore it's critical to collaborate with a healthcare provider who is aware of your particular requirements. In spite of the obstacles presented by Parkinson's disease, we may strengthen ourselves and nurture our bodies together to grow.

Chapter 7: Exercise and Physical Activity for Polycystic Kidney Disease

Benefits of Exercise for Polycystic Kidney Disease

1. Improved Cardiovascular Health:

The heightened risk of cardiovascular problems is one of the main worries for people with Parkinson's disease (PKD). An increased risk of heart disease and stroke can result from high blood pressure caused by kidney cyst development. Frequent exercise has been demonstrated to successfully lower the likelihood of these issues, thereby improving cardiovascular health. Exercises that increase cardiac muscle strength and blood circulation while lowering cholesterol include swimming and aerobic exercises. Because they ease the burden on the kidneys, these gains in cardiovascular health not only strengthen the heart but also promote renal health.

2. Reduced Blood Pressure:

Hypertension, or high blood pressure, is frequently linked to Parkinson's disease (PKD). Those who have the illness must effectively control their blood pressure in order to stop further kidney damage. One of the best methods for managing and lowering high blood pressure is exercise. Engaging in physical activity increases blood flow, blood vessel flexibility, and cardiovascular system efficiency. This slows the progression of PKD by lowering blood pressure and lessening the load on the kidneys.

3. Enhanced Mood and Mental Well-being:

PKD is a chronic illness that can have a negative impact on a person's mental health. Anxiety, depression, and a lower quality of life might result from the disease's physical and psychological stress. Thankfully, research has shown that exercise is a useful strategy for improving mood and fostering mental health. The "feel-good" hormones called endorphins are released by our brains when we exercise. These endorphins have a calming effect, increase mood, and enhance mental wellness in general. As a result, regular exercise can be an effective coping mechanism for people with Parkinson's disease (PKD), assisting them in overcoming the emotional obstacles that frequently accompany the illness.

4. Weight Management:

It is imperative for patients diagnosed with PKD to maintain a healthy weight, as obesity may worsen the disease's course and raise the possibility of complications. Frequent exercise is essential for weight management since it increases metabolism, burns calories, and builds lean muscle mass. Participating in exercises like cycling, strength training, or brisk walking can help you lose weight and keep it off. Furthermore, exercise helps control hunger and lessen cravings, which makes it simpler for people with PKD to adhere to a healthy diet and reach their weight objectives.

5. Improved Bone Strength:

Additionally, PKD can affect bone health, which can result in diseases like osteoporosis. Mineral balances, including those of calcium and phosphorus, which are critical for strong bones, might be upset by a decline in renal function. For the purpose of increasing bone strength and density, regular weight-bearing exercise, such as walking, running, or weightlifting, is essential. By putting stress on the bones, these activities encourage the body to produce more bone tissue and mineral density. In those with Parkinson's disease (PKD), strengthening the bones can lower the chance of fractures and improve overall skeletal health.

6. Enhanced Kidney Function:

Exercise on its own cannot reverse the progressive nature of kidney disease (PKD), but it can nevertheless improve kidney function. Regular exercise has been demonstrated to improve blood circulation and lower inflammation, which improve kidney function. Additionally, it aids in the management of diseases like obesity and diabetes that might exacerbate Parkinson's disease (PKD). Exercise helps to maintain general health and well-being, which in turn helps to better manage renal disease.

7. Increased Energy Levels:

One of the most prevalent symptoms that people with PKD have is fatigue. Living with the illness can take a toll on one's body and mind, which can deplete energy and make daily tasks difficult. By increasing energy and enhancing general stamina, adding exercise to a daily regimen can help fight fatigue. Frequent exercise increases lung capacity, fortifies the cardiovascular system, and builds muscle endurance, all of which help people feel more energised and more capable of doing everyday chores.

8. Social Engagement and Support:

People with Parkinson's disease (PKD) can interact with people who have experienced similar things by exercising on a regular basis. A sense of community can be created by enrolling in group fitness programmes or support groups, where people can share their stories, find emotional support, and gain insightful knowledge and coping mechanisms. Exercise's social component can help fight feelings of loneliness and provide people with Parkinson's disease (PKD) more confidence to take control of their health and wellbeing.

To sum up, exercise is essential to the treatment of polycystic kidney disease. The advantages of regular exercise are indisputable, ranging from elevating mood and fostering general well-being to lowering blood pressure and strengthening cardiovascular health. People with PKD can maintain their kidney health, enhance their quality of life, and take charge of their path to holistic well-being by including physical exercise into their daily routines.

Types of Exercise for Polycystic Kidney Disease

A healthy lifestyle is crucial for controlling Polycystic Kidney Disease (PKD), and exercise plays a major role in this. Exercise on a regular basis has been shown to improve cardiovascular health, enhance general well-being, aid in weight management, and lower the chance of acquiring several PKD-related problems. But not every kind of exercise is good for those with Parkinson's disease. It's critical to comprehend the various forms of exercise that can help people with Parkinson's disease (PKD) and how to include them in an all-encompassing exercise programme.

Aerobic Exercise:

Any activity that increases your heart rate and maintains it there for a prolonged amount of time is considered aerobic exercise, sometimes referred to as cardio exercise. This kind of exercise enhances circulation, fortifies the heart and lungs, and aids in maintaining a healthy weight. Frequent aerobic exercise can help PKD patients maintain better overall fitness levels, lower blood pressure, and lessen their risk of cardiovascular disease.

PKD patients can benefit from cardiovascular activity in a variety of ways, such as brisk walking, jogging, swimming, cycling, dancing, and using cardio equipment like treadmills or ellipticals. These exercises can be adjusted to fit the fitness levels of each individual and can be done for at least 30 minutes most days of the week at a moderate intensity. To prevent overexertion or potential injury, it's crucial to begin cautiously and increase the length and intensity of aerobic activity gradually.

Strength Training:

To develop and tone your muscles, strength training, sometimes referred to as resistance training, uses weights, resistance bands, or your own body weight. Patients with Parkinson's disease (PKD) can benefit from strength training since it can enhance muscle strength and endurance, preserve bone density, and support healthy joints. Strength exercise can also support a healthy metabolism and help with weight management.

PKD patients can engage in strength training activities two to three times per week, focusing on all major muscle groups. Exercises like lunges, push-ups, bicep curls, and shoulder presses can be a part of this. It's crucial to begin with modest weights and increase resistance and intensity gradually as you develop strength and stamina. It is highly encouraged to get help from a skilled trainer or therapist since proper form and technique are essential in preventing injuries.

Flexibility Exercises:

Increased muscular flexibility and joint range of motion are the main goals of flexibility exercises. These exercises can aid in easing stiffness in the muscles, enhancing mobility overall, and improving posture. Flexibility exercises can be very useful for PKD patients in reducing pain and suffering related to cyst growth.

Patients with Parkinson's disease can benefit from flexibility activities such as yoga, tai chi, Pilates, and stretching. All of the main muscle groups are targeted by these workouts, which can be done regularly. Before beginning any flexibility exercises, it's crucial to warm up and concentrate on calm, deliberate motions to minimise overstretching. As with any exercise, it's crucial to pay attention to your body's demands and limitations and adjust activities as necessary.

Low-Impact Activities:

Exercises that are low-impact are kinder to the body and place less strain on the joints. Because they lower the danger of harm and lessen the pressure on the kidneys, these exercises are especially advantageous for people with Parkinson's disease (PKD). Muscle strength, cardiovascular health, and general fitness can all be enhanced by low-impact exercise.

Low-impact exercises that can be beneficial for persons with Parkinson's disease (PKD) include swimming, water aerobics, cycling, utilising an elliptical machine, and rowing. These exercises minimise the strain on the joints while offering a cardiovascular workout. It's crucial to begin with shorter workouts and build up to longer and more intense ones as your fitness level rises. In order to prevent strain or injury, it's also critical to maintain correct form and technique.

Finding the Right Balance:

It's crucial to strike the ideal balance when it comes to fitness and your lifestyle as a patient with PKD. It's critical to pay attention to your body and recognise your limits in order to avoid overdoing it and any consequences. Several important factors to take into account while creating your workout regimen are:

1. Consulting with a healthcare provider: See your healthcare professional before to beginning any fitness programme, particularly if you have any pre-existing conditions or concerns. They can offer advice and assist you in creating a customised fitness programme that takes into consideration your unique requirements and constraints.

2. Gradually increasing intensity and duration: It's crucial to begin cautiously and increase the duration and intensity of your workouts over time. In addition to allowing your body to adjust, this helps you avoid overdoing it and getting hurt. It's critical to pay attention to your body and adjust your exercises to fit your specific requirements.

3. Monitoring your symptoms: Observe closely how your body reacts to physical activity. It's critical to take a step back and modify your exercise regimen if you feel any pain, discomfort, or strange sensations during or after your workout. It's crucial to drink plenty of water and to stop frequently as needed.

4. Incorporating rest and recovery: Exercise alone is not as crucial as rest and recuperation. To give your body time to repair and regenerate, remember to include rest days in your workout regimen.

This can support general wellbeing and aid in the prevention of overuse injuries.

5. Seeking guidance from a professional: It could be helpful to get advice from a trained professional if you are new to exercising or if you have certain restrictions or concerns. They may offer you individualised advice and assist you in developing a fitness regimen that is both efficient and safe for you.

To sum up, physical activity plays a critical role in the management of polycystic kidney disease. Patients with Parkinson's disease (PKD) can benefit specifically from aerobic exercise, weight training, flexibility exercises, and low-impact activities. A customised workout plan that meets your needs and enhances general wellbeing requires finding the perfect balance and paying attention to your body. You may maintain a healthy weight, strengthen your cardiovascular system, and improve your general quality of life by making exercise a part of your daily routine.

Precautions and Modifications for Exercise in Polycystic Kidney Disease

Exercise and physical activity present special obstacles for those with polycystic kidney disease (PKD). Kidney cysts can cause pain, discomfort, and other symptoms that can make it difficult for the patient to do specific physical activities. I have worked with numerous PKD patients as a physician and health and wellness coach, and I have seen the positive effects of exercise on their general health and wellbeing. When it comes to exercise, it is important for people with PKD to be aware of their limitations and adopt the necessary safety measures.

Speaking with a medical expert, particularly a nephrologist or renal specialist with experience treating PKD patients, is one of the first and most crucial steps in creating an exercise programme for these individuals. These experts will be able to offer customised counsel and direction in light of the patient's unique situation and any difficulties they could be dealing with. They may answer any worries or inquiries the patient may have in addition to assisting in determining the safe and suitable amount of physical exercise.

Patients with Parkinson's disease (PKD) should listen to their bodies and notice any symptoms or pain that may emerge while exercise once medical clearance has been received. Urinary tract infections and soreness or discomfort in the lower back or abdomen are common in people with Parkinson's disease (PKD). It is imperative that you report these symptoms to a healthcare provider right away and avoid ignoring them.

Certain adjustments to the workout regimen could be required to reduce the chance of injury or symptom worsening. For instance, high-impact exercises or abrupt direction changes, such sprinting or jumping, may need to be avoided or adjusted. Low-impact activities like swimming, cycling, or walking might be more appropriate for people with Parkinson's disease.

Patients with Parkinson's disease (PKD) may potentially benefit from strength training activities since they enhance muscle strength and general physical function. But be careful when doing these exercises—using large weights or putting too much effort on the kidneys might cause more damage. It is crucial to begin with modest weights and increase the intensity progressively as tolerated, all while being supervised by a licenced strength and conditioning consultant or medical professional.

Patients with Parkinson's disease (PKD) should adjust not only the kind and level of exercise they perform, but also the time and length of their exercises. Instead of planning a single, lengthy workout, it might be necessary to organise shorter, more regular workouts throughout the day. By doing so, the chance of overexertion and symptom exacerbation can be reduced.

Staying well hydrated is crucial when exercising for persons with Parkinson's disease. Drinking enough water is essential for people with PKD because it keeps the kidneys functioning and helps flush out toxins. To avoid being dehydrated and to maintain healthy kidney function, it is advised to consume water before to, during, and following physical activity. On the other hand, as some people with PKD may have negative effects from excessive fluid consumption, it is crucial to speak with a healthcare provider regarding the right amount of fluid intake.

Patients with Parkinson's disease (PKD) may benefit from adding other lifestyle changes to their daily regimen in addition to exercising. These could include altering one's nutrition, learning stress-reduction strategies, and keeping a healthy weight. It is crucial to collaborate with a registered dietitian or other healthcare provider to create a meal plan that is customised to each person's unique requirements and tastes. This could entail consuming less sodium, eating more fruits and vegetables, and keeping an eye on how much protein you consume.

Stress management should also be a top priority for PKD patients because it might impair kidney function. Numerous self-help methods, including deep breathing exercises, relaxation training, and meditation, can help lower stress levels and improve general wellbeing.

For people with Parkinson's disease (PKD), maintaining a healthy body weight is especially essential because being overweight might exacerbate renal strain. A balanced diet and regular exercise can assist people with Parkinson's disease (PKD) in reaching and maintaining a healthy weight. But it's crucial to handle weight control carefully because extreme exercise regimens or crash diets might harm kidney function. For individualised advice, it is always advised to speak with a licenced dietician or other healthcare provider.

To sum up, physical activity has the potential to be an effective means of controlling polycystic kidney disease (PKD) and enhancing general health and wellness. Exercise should be approached cautiously by people with PKD, and any necessary adjustments should be made in light of their unique symptoms and condition. Key actions in guaranteeing a safe and successful exercise programme for people with Parkinson's disease (PKD) include speaking with a healthcare provider, keeping an eye on symptoms, and modifying the exercise regimen as needed. Patients with Parkinson's disease (PKD) can take charge of their health and enhance their quality of life by making exercise and other lifestyle changes part of their daily routine.

Incorporating Physical Activity Into Daily Life With Polycystic Kidney Disease

Being physically active is crucial for leading a happy and healthy life, especially for those who have polycystic kidney disease (PKD). Frequent exercise can help control symptoms, enhance general health, and lower the chance of complications related to Parkinson's disease. But managing physical activity in daily life can be difficult for people with Parkinson's disease. I'll give you some useful advice in this subsection to assist you get through these obstacles and incorporate physical activity into your daily routine in a sustainable way.

Overcoming potential obstacles is a crucial first step towards integrating physical activity into your everyday life if you have Parkinson's disease (PKD). A few typical obstacles are discomfort, exhaustion, injury fear, and the impression that there isn't enough time. To create a practical and doable workout regimen, it's critical to recognise and overcome these obstacles.

It's important to pay attention to your body and begin with activities that suit your current energy level if you want to overcome weariness. This can entail beginning with low-impact workouts like swimming or walking and progressively upping the intensity as your energy levels rise. Finding the right balance between pushing oneself to the limit and not overdoing it is crucial since overdoing it can exacerbate existing pain and exhaustion.

Since kidney inflammation and discomfort can result from kidney cysts, pain is another major obstacle for people with PKD. Before beginning any workout programme, it's crucial to speak with your medical team to be sure you're doing things that are safe for your condition. They could suggest particular workouts that might assist reduce discomfort and enhance the condition of the kidneys. For instance, doing mild stretching exercises can assist the muscles that surround the kidneys become more flexible and less tense.

Another possible obstacle that can keep people with PKD from exercising is their fear of getting hurt. This concern might be warranted because engaging in some high-impact activities raises the possibility of kidney damage or cyst rupture. This does not imply, however, that any physical exercise has to be avoided. It's critical to collaborate closely with your medical team to determine the kinds of activities that are appropriate and safe for your condition. They might suggest low-impact workouts like tai chi, yoga, or cycling since they have many health advantages without placing an excessive amount of strain on the kidneys.

Regardless of their health, a typical hurdle for many people is a perceived lack of time. Finding time for exercise, however, is essential for controlling Parkinson's disease and preserving general health. It's critical to understand that physical activity doesn't have to be difficult or time-consuming. Engaging in brief spurts of physical activity throughout the day can accumulate and yield substantial health advantages. You can increase your level of physical activity by doing things like walking during your lunch break, using the stairs instead of the elevator, and spending a few minutes each morning stretching.

After overcoming these obstacles, it's critical to establish reasonable objectives for integrating exercise into your everyday routine. Setting attainable goals is crucial to keeping up motivation and sticking to a workout schedule. Find enjoyable things that you can still participate in at your present level of fitness. If you want to swim, for instance, you may try to go swimming three times a week for thirty minutes each time. Establishing objectives that are clear, quantifiable, doable, pertinent, and time-bound is crucial (SMART). You may monitor your development and maintain motivation by doing this.

Finding hobbies and pursuits that suit your interests and preferences is also crucial. You are more likely to persist in your hobbies over time when you find them enjoyable. Engaging in physical activity should be enjoyable and fulfilling rather than a work. This could entail experimenting with various pursuits and investigating various workout choices until you discover something that speaks to you. It could be anything at all, like taking up gardening, dancing, or playing sports. Try out various hobbies and pay attention to your body's signals to determine what suits you the best.

Finding things you can stick with over time is another requirement for incorporating physical activity into your daily life. Selecting pursuits that you can see yourself engaging in for the long term and that fit into your lifestyle is crucial. Having a range of activities in your routine is also beneficial since it can keep you from getting bored and offer a variety of mental and physical challenges. This could entail combining several exercise modalities, such as aerobic, strength, and flexibility training, to develop a comprehensive fitness regimen that targets all facets of fitness.

To sum up, it is critical for general health and wellbeing with Parkinson's disease (PKD) to include physical activity in daily life. You can incorporate physical activity into your routine in a sustainable way by overcoming obstacles, establishing reasonable goals, and engaging in fun activities. Prior to beginning any fitness regimen, get advice from your healthcare provider, and pay attention to your body as you go. By being committed and persistent, you can use exercise as a tool to control your Parkinson's disease and lead a better, more satisfying life.

Chapter 8: Managing Pain and Discomfort in Polycystic Kidney Disease

Understanding Pain in Polycystic Kidney Disease

Among the most concerning symptoms that people with polycystic kidney disease (PKD) encounter is frequently pain. It can manifest in different forms and has a significant effect on a person's quality of life. Maintaining general health and wellbeing requires an understanding of the various forms of pain associated with Parkinson's disease (PKD) and appropriate management of that pain.

Abdominal discomfort is one of the most prevalent forms of pain that people with PKD encounter. The growth of kidney cysts usually causes pressure and straining of the surrounding organs and tissues, which is the cause of this pain. Though it can occasionally be intense and piercing, the pain is typically described as dull and achy. The pain may be intermittent or continuous, and its intensity ranges from mild to severe.

Another form of pain that people with PKD may encounter is flank pain. Usually, the sides of the abdomen, directly below the ribs, are the location of this ache. Many people describe it as a sharp, stabbing pain that gets worse when they move or engage in physical activity. The swelling of the kidneys and the pressure they put on the surrounding tissues can induce flank discomfort, which varies in severity and duration.

Urinary discomfort is a common symptom of Parkinson's disease (PKD), in addition to flank and abdominal pain. This pain, which is usually described as scorching or stinging, is usually experienced during urination. Other symptoms of the urinary tract, like urgency, frequency, and blood in the urine, may accompany it. Because PKD patients have aberrant kidney structure and function, urinary tract infections and stones are more common in this population and can cause urinary pain.

Pain in people with Parkinson's disease (PKD) can have many different origins, thus in order to create a suitable care strategy, it's critical to precisely pinpoint the underlying reasons of the pain. The following are typical PKD causes of pain:

1. Cyst enlargement: Cysts can strain on surrounding tissues and organs as they enlarge, causing pain.

2. Kidney stone formation: Kidney stones can be extremely painful when they move through the urinary tract, and people with PKD are more likely to acquire kidney stones.

3. Urinary tract infections: Urinary tract infections can be painful and uncomfortable, and they are more common in people with Parkinson's disease (PKD).

4. Hemorrhage or rupture of cysts: Kidney cysts can occasionally bleed or burst, resulting in abrupt, excruciating agony.

5. Inflammation: Nephritis, or kidney inflammation, can be painful and uncomfortable.

Precisely determining the fundamental sources of discomfort in Parkinson's disease is essential for efficient handling. Imaging tests, such ultrasounds, CT scans, or MRIs, can assist determine the existence of kidney stones, examine the size and location of cysts, and rule out other possible causes of pain.

A thorough management strategy can be created once the underlying source of pain has been identified. To give comprehensive pain management, this plan may involve a mix of complementary therapies, lifestyle changes, and medicinal measures. PKD pain treatment techniques could involve:

1. Medications: Mild to moderate pain can be reduced using over-the-counter painkillers, such as nonsteroidal anti-inflammatory medications (NSAIDs). Prescription drugs like opioids or muscle relaxants could be required in extreme situations.

2. Lifestyle modifications: Maintaining a healthy lifestyle can aid with pain management and wellbeing enhancement. This can entail

maintaining a healthy diet, working out frequently, controlling stress, and getting enough relaxation and sleep.

3. Complementary therapies: Acupuncture, massage, and relaxation techniques are a few examples of complementary therapies that can help relieve pain further and enhance general relaxation and wellbeing.

4. Cyst management: To ease pain and stop more issues, cysts may need to be surgically removed or drained. Usually, this kind of intervention is limited to people who have sizable cysts that cause symptoms.

5. Urinary tract infection management: Appropriate antibiotic treatment is required to eradicate urinary tract infections and relieve symptoms if they are causing pain.

Keep in mind that there is no one-size-fits-all method for managing pain in people with Parkinson's disease. Every person may experience pain differently and react differently to different interventions. To create a customised pain management plan, close collaboration with a medical practitioner, nephrologist, and pain management specialist is necessary.

In summary, maintaining general health and wellbeing in the context of polycystic kidney disease requires an understanding of and ability to manage discomfort. The various forms of pain that people with Parkinson's disease (PKD) may endure, including flank, abdominal, and urinary pain, can significantly affect their quality of life. To effectively relieve pain and enhance overall wellbeing, it is crucial to accurately diagnose the underlying causes of pain and to adopt a comprehensive management strategy that incorporates lifestyle changes, medical procedures, and complementary therapies. People with Parkinson's disease (PKD) can improve their quality of life and recover control over their lives by adopting a comprehensive strategy to pain management.

Medications for Pain Management in Polycystic Kidney Disease

Adopting a multimodal approach that integrates many tactics is essential for achieving optimal outcomes when it comes to pain management in Parkinson's disease (PKD). For people with PKD, medications are crucial to reducing discomfort and enhancing quality of life. Medication, it is crucial to remember, is only one component of the puzzle and should be utilised in concert with other holistic methods, including coping mechanisms, food planning, counselling, psychology-related tactics, self-care substitutes, counselling, and lifestyle modifications.

In PKD, analgesics—also referred to as painkillers—are frequently the primary line of treatment for pain management. These drugs relieve patients' pain by obstructing the body's natural process of transmitting pain signals. Non-opioid and opioid analgesics are the two primary categories of analgesics.

When treating mild to moderate pain, non-opioid analgesics like acetaminophen are frequently the first to be used. When used as prescribed, acetaminophen, commonly referred to as paracetamol, is generally safe and readily available over-the-counter. It functions by preventing the brain's generation of certain chemicals that result in fever and pain. But since taking too much acetaminophen might harm the liver, it's crucial to abide by the suggested dosage recommendations and not go over the daily maximum.

Even though acetaminophen is usually safe, it is important to speak with a doctor before using any medicine to treat pain in Parkinson's disease. This is due to the fact that PKD can have an adverse effect on the kidneys, and people with CKD may need to use some analgesics, including acetaminophen, with caution (Chronic Kidney Disease).

Opioid analgesics may be prescribed when non-opioid analgesics are insufficient. Opioids, which include morphine, oxycodone, and codeine, function by attaching themselves to particular receptors in the brain and spinal cord and preventing the transmission of pain signals. These drugs are stronger and have the potential to significantly reduce pain, particularly in cases of extreme discomfort. To reduce the risk of adverse effects and dependence, opioids must be administered under strict medical supervision due to their potent effects on the central nervous system.

Although analgesics are useful in the management of pain, it's crucial to understand that they might only offer momentary respite. In addition, prolonged usage of opioids can result in addiction, dependency, and tolerance. In order to choose the best course of action for your unique circumstances, it is imperative that you investigate alternative approaches to pain management and collaborate closely with a medical practitioner.

In PKD, nonsteroidal anti-inflammatory medicines (NSAIDs) are another class of treatments that are frequently used to alleviate pain. These drugs assist in lowering inflammation and easing discomfort brought on by irritated organs or tissues. NSAIDs function by preventing the synthesis of prostaglandins, which are substances that increase fever, discomfort, and inflammation.

Over-the-counter medications called nonsteroidal anti-inflammatory drugs (NSAIDs), such ibuprofen and naproxen, are useful in treating mild to moderate pain. These drugs can impact kidney function, therefore it's important to use them carefully in people with PKD. NSAIDs cause the kidneys' blood arteries to narrow, which can exacerbate renal function in people whose kidney health is already damaged and lower blood flow to the kidneys.

Those who have Parkinson's disease (PKD) should speak with a doctor before using NSAIDs to treat pain. They will evaluate your kidney function and work with you to decide if NSAIDs are a good choice for you. In rare circumstances, they might suggest less risky pain relief techniques for your kidneys.

For the purpose of managing pain in Parkinson's disease, additional painkillers may be used in addition to analgesics and nonsteroidal antidepressants. These consist of muscle relaxants, antidepressants, anticonvulsants, and topical drugs.

Anticonvulsants, including pregabalin and gabapentin, are drugs that are frequently used to treat seizures, but they can also be useful in lowering neuropathic pain. Because the cysts squeeze the nerves, PKD patients may frequently experience neuropathic pain, which is pain brought on by destruction or malfunction of the nervous system. Anticonvulsants function by lessening the transmission of pain signals and stabilising overexcited neurons.

Antidepressants, especially tricyclic antidepressants such as amitriptyline, have been shown to be helpful in the treatment of Parkinson's disease pain. These drugs function in two ways: they block the central nervous system from transmitting pain signals and raise the amounts of specific chemicals in the brain that aid in mood regulation.

Pain from the muscle spasms that are typical in Parkinson's disease (PKD) can be managed with the use of muscle relaxants like baclofen or tizanidine. These drugs function by easing tense muscles and preventing pain signals from the muscles from reaching the brain.

Topical treatments, including creams or patches containing lidocaine, can be placed directly to the skin over the injured region to relieve pain in that specific location. These drugs function by numbing the skin's nerves and preventing the pain signals from being transmitted.

The best drugs and treatment strategy for your particular needs must be decided in close consultation with your physician or a pain management specialist. The intensity of your pain, any possible adverse effects, and any conflicts with other medications you might be taking are just a few of the variables they will take into account.

In summary, drugs are essential for controlling pain in Parkinson's disease. They should, therefore, be combined with other holistic methods like coping mechanisms, food planning, counselling, psychology-related procedures, self-care substitutes, and self-help methods. It's critical to keep in mind that drugs have hazards and side effects in addition to providing momentary respite. Therefore, for best outcomes in raising the quality of life for people with Parkinson's disease (PKD), it is imperative to collaborate closely with a healthcare provider and investigate a multimodal strategy to pain treatment.

Non-Pharmacological Pain Management Techniques for Polycystic Kidney Disease

Persistent discomfort is among the most typical symptoms that people with polycystic kidney disease (PKD) encounter. The intensity and debilitating nature of chronic pain can vary, negatively impacting the quality of life for those who experience it. In addition to pharmaceuticals, non-pharmacological methods can be utilised as adjunctive therapies to effectively control pain.

To ease the pain associated with Parkinson's disease (PKD), heat therapy is a straightforward and efficient method. Heat has the ability to ease muscle tension, enhance blood flow, and lessen inflammation in the afflicted areas. Heat therapy can be used in a number of ways, such as with hot packs, warm baths, or even hot water bottles. You can temporarily relieve the affected area and enhance overall comfort by applying heat for a duration of 15 to 20 minutes.

Unlike heat therapy, cold therapy can also be helpful in treating discomfort associated with Parkinson's disease. Cold therapy acts by numbing the affected area, decreasing inflammation, and narrowing blood vessels. Cold therapy can be used with ice packs, cool compresses, or cold showers. It's crucial to cover ice packs when applying them to avoid making direct contact with the skin, which can lead to injury. For ten to fifteen minutes, cold therapy can be applied to relieve pain and suffering.

Another non-pharmacological pain management strategy that can assist people with Parkinson's disease (PKD) in managing their symptoms is relaxation training. Deep breathing, progressive muscle relaxation, and guided imagery are a few examples of relaxation techniques that can ease tension in the muscles and help people feel less stressed. These workouts are very accessible and convenient because they may be performed anytime and anyplace. People with PKD can significantly reduce their pain and feel better about themselves by adding relaxation techniques into their daily routine.

Distraction methods work well for treating pain associated with Parkinson's disease. People with Parkinson's disease (PKD) are less likely to feel pain when they are involved in an activity that focuses and holds their attention. Engaging in hobbies or artistic pursuits, reading, watching movies, or listening to music are examples of distraction tactics. People with PKD may notice a reduction in the severity of their pain and an increase in their mood by focusing their attention on something entertaining or engaging instead of their discomfort.

It is crucial to remember that non-pharmacological pain relief methods shouldn't take the place of prescription drugs from medical professionals. These methods are designed to give people with Parkinson's disease (PKD) more relief in addition to medical treatment. Before beginning any new pain management methods, it is advised to speak with a healthcare professional to be sure they are safe and suitable for your particular situation.

In summary, non-pharmacological pain relief methods can be effective instruments for treating pain associated with Parkinson's disease. Immediate alleviation, inflammation reduction, relaxation, and overall well-being can be achieved through the use of heat therapy, cold therapy, relaxation exercises, and distraction tactics. People with Parkinson's disease (PKD) can actively participate in controlling their symptoms and enhancing their quality of life by adopting these strategies into their everyday routine. Always get medical advice before beginning any new pain management measures to make sure they are appropriate for your requirements and situation.

References:

1. Research study: A Systematic Review of Heat Therapy for Chronic Pain. Journal of Complementary & Alternative Medicine.

2. Research study: Cold Therapy for Pain: An Analysis of Previous Research. The Pain Management Journal.

3. Research study: Relaxation Techniques for Chronic Pain Management: An Organized Review. The Holistic Nursing Journal.

4. Research study: Distraction Techniques for Pain Management: A Comprehensive Analysis. The Pain Management Journal.

Seeking Medical Care for Pain in Polycystic Kidney Disease

One of the most prevalent symptoms of polycystic kidney disease is pain (PKD). It can impact many people' quality of life and range from minor discomfort to severe and persistent pain. As a physician with a focus on holistic medicine and a health and wellness coach, I know how critical it is to address pain management requirements holistically. This subchapter will provide information on how to get medical attention for pain in people with Parkinson's disease (PKD), with a focus on advocacy, open communication, and looking into non-traditional treatment alternatives.

Honest and open communication with medical providers is essential when it comes to treating pain in people with Parkinson's disease. It's critical for patients to communicate their worries, describe the type and intensity of their pain, and describe how it interferes with their everyday activities. Effective pain management in people with Parkinson's disease (PKD) requires open communication with your healthcare team. Treatments for pain can vary based on the underlying reasons and specific needs of each patient.

People with Parkinson's disease (PKD) may feel a variety of pains, from acute to chronic. Acute pain is frequently brief, abrupt, and brought on by a specific event, such as an infection or kidney stone. Conversely, chronic pain is ongoing and may occur intermittently over a long length of time. Kidney stones, enlarged cysts, or other PKD problems may be the cause. Your healthcare team can choose the best course of action for you if they are aware of the kind and severity of your pain.

A crucial component of getting medical attention for pain in Parkinson's disease is advocacy. Advocating for your pain management requirements and actively participating in your own treatment is crucial. Communicating your objectives, concerns, and preferences to your healthcare staff is crucial. This includes talking about your pain threshold, any pain management techniques you've used in the past that worked for you, and any side effects or worries you may have regarding specific drugs. You can collaborate with your healthcare team to develop a customised treatment plan that meets your unique requirements and goals by taking an active role in your own pain management.

Examining complementary and alternative therapies can be helpful in addition to conventional medical methods for the management of pain in Parkinson's disease. It's critical to keep an open mind and take alternative therapies into consideration. As a health and wellness coach, I frequently suggest to my PKD patients dietary and lifestyle planning, counselling, psychology-related approaches, alternative and complementary forms of self-care, self-help methods, and coping mechanisms. These methods concentrate on raising holistic health, lowering stress levels, and enhancing general well-being.

Changes in lifestyle can have a big impact on how well people with Parkinson's disease (PKD) manage their discomfort and stay healthy overall. Regular exercise, such swimming or low-impact walking, can aid with pain relief, circulation improvement, and muscle strengthening. Aside from minimising discomfort, dietary modifications like drinking more water and consuming less salt can help improve kidney function. Furthermore, by encouraging relaxation and easing physical tension, stress-reduction methods like yoga, deep breathing exercises, and meditation can aid in the management of pain.

Pain-stricken PKD patients may potentially benefit from counselling and psychology-related interventions. Feelings of irritation, worry, and despair can result from chronic pain, which can have a substantial negative influence on mental health and wellbeing. Consulting a psychologist or counsellor for therapeutic support can offer coping mechanisms and stress-reduction techniques, as well as enhance one's mental health in general.

Complementary and alternative methods of self-care can be included into a complete plan for managing Parkinson's disease pain. These could consist of herbal medicines, heat or cold therapy, massage therapy, and acupuncture. These alternative techniques help many people find healing and greater well-being, while individual results may vary in their effectiveness. It is crucial to communicate any alternative treatments you are thinking about to your healthcare team, though, as they might interfere with prescription drugs or be inadvisable for some PKD patients.

Coping mechanisms and self-help approaches are also useful tools for pain management in Parkinson's disease. These might include writing, mindfulness meditation, deep breathing exercises, and partaking in joyful pursuits that detach from suffering. Joining networks or support groups for people with Parkinson's disease (PKD) can also foster a feeling of belonging and understanding by facilitating the exchange of experiences, counsel, and emotional support.

In summary, getting the right medical care for pain in Parkinson's disease (PKD) necessitates being upfront with medical staff, speaking up for the needs of pain management, and looking for alternate therapy choices. You can collaborate with your healthcare team to create a customised pain management plan by talking about the type and intensity of your pain, communicating your preferences and concerns, and actively engaging in your own treatment. Furthermore, investigating other modalities—such as coping mechanisms, counselling and psychology-related approaches, substitutes for self-care, and lifestyle adjustments—can enhance general wellbeing and offer extra support. Recall that there are tools and services available to assist you in managing your discomfort and leading a full life, and that you are not alone in your journey with Parkinson's disease.

Chapter 9: Managing High Blood Pressure in Polycystic Kidney Disease

Understanding the Link Between Polycystic Kidney Disease and High Blood Pressure

Subchapter 5.1: The Connection Unveiled

Throughout my career, I have treated innumerable individuals with polycystic kidney disease (PKD) as a medical practitioner and health and wellness coach. One of the most prevalent issues I encounter is the elevated blood pressure that frequently occurs in people with Parkinson's disease (PKD). The purpose of this subchapter is to clarify the relationship between these two circumstances and how they affect one another. Gaining a thorough understanding of this relationship will enable us to take more control over our health.

Multiple renal cyst development is a hallmark of the complicated hereditary disease known as PKD. Over time, these cysts expand gradually, causing the kidneys to enlarge and function less well. Although PKD primarily affects the kidneys, it can also have an impact on the cardiovascular system and other systems in the body.

Elevated blood pressure is a defining feature of high blood pressure, sometimes referred to as hypertension. It is a prevalent comorbidity that affects roughly 60–70% of patients with Parkinson's disease (PKD). It's interesting to note that elevated blood pressure may also serve as a marker for the severity and advancement of PKD.

What connection exists, then, between PKD and hypertension? The complex interactions between renal cysts and the cardiovascular system hold the key to the solution. The renal arteries, which carry blood to the kidneys, may become abnormally shaped or function abnormally due to cysts in Parkinson's disease. This may cause a number of physiological alterations, which in turn may raise blood pressure.

Subchapter 5.2: The Role of Renin-Angiotensin-Aldosterone System (RAAS)

In order to comprehend the process by which PKD leads to hypertension, we need to examine the function of the Renin-Angiotensin-Aldosterone System (RAAS). The hormone system known as the RAAS controls the body's fluid balance and blood pressure. It is made up of renin, angiotensin, and aldosterone, among other essential ingredients.

Renin is the enzyme that converts angiotensinogen to angiotensin I, and kidney cysts in people with PKD can increase this enzyme's synthesis. After then, angiotensin I is changed into angiotensin II, a strong vasoconstrictor that causes blood vessels to narrow and blood pressure to rise. Angiotensin II also causes the release of aldosterone, a hormone that encourages the kidneys to retain water and salt, which raises blood pressure even further.

In addition to impairing normal blood pressure regulation, RAAS activation in PKD also negatively impacts renal function. Renal fibrosis, which is typified by the buildup of too much connective tissue in the kidneys, can result from prolonged RAAS activation. Renal fibrosis aggravates the course of Parkinson's disease and deteriorates kidney function even more.

Subchapter 5.3: Consequences for Kidney Function

The way high blood pressure and Parkinson's disease interact has a big impact on kidney function. High blood pressure can cause cyst walls to compress, which can enlarge the cysts and cause them to secrete more fluid. This then deteriorates the kidneys' ability to filter and excrete substances, further harming healthy kidney tissue.

In addition, the increased pressure inside the cysts may cause intracystic haemorrhages or ruptures. These occurrences cause the cysts to leak blood, which inflames the area and encourages the formation of new cysts. The ongoing cycle of cyst development and growth exacerbates the impairment of renal function.

Furthermore, in people with PKD, long-term high blood pressure can cause chronic kidney injury. Plaque accumulation in the arteries is known as atherosclerosis, a condition that can be brought on by persistently high blood pressure. Further renal damage results from compromised blood supply to the kidneys caused by atherosclerosis-related narrowing or blockage of the renal arteries.

Subchapter 5.4: The Importance of Blood Pressure Management

Considering the complex interrelationship between hypertension and Parkinson's disease (PKD), it is clear that controlling blood pressure well is essential to the overall therapy of PKD. The development of problems and the rate at which kidney damage progresses can both be slowed down with proper blood pressure monitoring and management.

In my practise, I place a strong emphasis on managing blood pressure holistically. I work with my patients to make lifestyle adjustments, like as eating a balanced diet, exercising regularly, reducing stress, and getting adequate sleep, in addition to standard drugs. Blood pressure management and general well-being may be significantly impacted by these lifestyle modifications.

In addition, routine blood pressure monitoring is necessary to identify hypertension in people with PKD early on. This enables prompt intervention and the start of suitable treatment plans to stop more kidney damage.

Subchapter 5.5: Coping Strategies and Self-Care Techniques

It might be difficult to manage high blood pressure and PKD on a physical and emotional level. In order to improve their general well-being, people with chronic disorders must learn coping mechanisms and self-care practises.

Learning about the illnesses and getting help from medical professionals, support groups, or internet communities are two useful coping mechanisms. It can be reassuring and empowering to share information and experiences with people going through comparable struggles.

Self-care methods can help lower stress levels and improve general wellness. Examples of these methods include mindfulness exercises, deep breathing exercises, and relaxation techniques. Positivity and better well-being can also be facilitated by partaking in joyful and fulfilling activities, such hobbies or quality time with loved ones.

In conclusion, for efficient treatment and better results, it is essential to comprehend the connection between PKD and hypertension. Understanding the complex interactions among these disorders allows us to design focused approaches to manage blood pressure, maintain renal function, and improve health in general. With a comprehensive strategy that includes stress reduction, lifestyle adjustments, and self-care practises, we can empower ourselves to take charge of our health and live happy, meaningful lives in spite of these obstacles.

Recall that you have the ability to handle your journey toward managing high blood pressure and PKD with grace and resilience.

Lifestyle Modifications for Blood Pressure Control in Polycystic Kidney Disease

Subchapter: Practical Tips for Making Lifestyle Modifications

Importance of Sodium Restriction

Being a physician with a focus on holistic healthcare and a health and wellness coach, I have personally witnessed the tremendous influence that lifestyle changes can have on blood pressure control in patients with polycystic kidney disease (PKD). I'll offer helpful advice on how to change your lifestyle in this subchapter to lower blood pressure in people with PKD. We will discuss the significance of stress management, frequent exercise, weight control, and sodium restriction.

Let's talk about the significance of sodium restriction first and foremost. Sodium is a necessary mineral that is critical to the fluid balance and neuronal function of our bodies. But taking too much salt can cause high blood pressure and fluid retention, which can worsen the problems of Parkinson's disease. People with PKD must be careful about how much sodium they eat.

Reducing your consumption of packaged and processed foods is one of the best strategies to cut back on salt. These goods frequently include large amounts of sodium that isn't readily apparent because of additives, taste enhancers, and preservatives. Choosing whole, fresh meals will help you cut back on sodium consumption considerably. Furthermore, adopting low-sodium substitutes and reading food labels can help lower blood pressure in those with PKD.

Reducing the amount of table salt you use and substituting it with other herbs and flavours is another useful suggestion for cutting back on sodium. This lowers the total amount of sodium in your diet while also giving your foods more flavour. You also have more control over the ingredients and sodium level of your meals when you prepare at home.

Weight Management

For general health and especially for controlling blood pressure in people with Parkinson's disease (PKD), maintaining a healthy weight is essential. Being overweight puts extra burden on the kidneys, which raises blood pressure. For people with PKD, it is crucial to reach and maintain a healthy weight.

Stressing the importance of eating a healthy, balanced diet is one of the main strategies for managing weight. You may stay at a healthy weight by including whole grains, lean proteins, fruits, vegetables, and healthy fats in your diet. It's also critical to watch portion sizes and refrain from overindulging.

Additionally, blood pressure control and weight management are significantly impacted by physical exercise. Frequent exercise enhances cardiovascular health in addition to helping with weight loss. Walking, swimming, cycling, and yoga are a few exercises that can help lower blood pressure and minimise the chance of having PKD problems. Always make sure it's safe for you to begin any fitness plan by speaking with your healthcare provider first.

Regular Exercise

Frequent exercise is beneficial for controlling blood pressure in people with Parkinson's disease (PKD) and is also essential for managing weight. Engaging in physical activity can strengthen the heart, enhance blood circulation, lower cholesterol, and lessen stress—all of which can lead to better control of blood pressure.

Aerobic activities that increase heart rate, including jogging, cycling, dancing, or brisk walking, can successfully lower blood pressure. Try to get in at least 150 minutes a week of moderate-to-intense aerobic activity or 75 minutes a week of strenuous aerobic activity. Furthermore, adding strength training activities two or three times a week might enhance blood pressure management and cardiovascular health even more.

It is imperative that you begin your workouts cautiously and build up to longer and more intense sessions. Recognize your limitations and pay attention to your body. Get medical help right away if you feel any pain or discomfort during exercising.

Stress Reduction

Let's now talk about the important influence that stress-reduction strategies can have on PKD patients' ability to control their blood pressure. Prolonged stress has been shown to increase blood pressure and exacerbate PKD symptoms. Thus, using stress-reduction strategies is essential for general wellbeing.

People with PKD can lower their stress levels in many different ways by implementing various strategies into their daily life. Tai chi, yoga, deep breathing techniques, and mindfulness meditation are a few instances. Finding time for self-care and participating in enjoyable hobbies are also crucial for reducing stress.

Recall that stress management is a lifetime habit, and it could take some time to figure out what suits you best. If you don't get results right away, don't give up. When used consistently and assiduously, stress-reduction strategies can be an effective means of controlling blood pressure and enhancing general health in people with Parkinson's disease.

Conclusion

In summary, changing one's lifestyle is essential for managing blood pressure in patients with polycystic kidney disease. People with PKD can greatly enhance their general health and well-being by adhering to the useful advice provided in this subchapter, which includes sodium limitation, weight management, regular exercise, and stress reduction. Recall that minor adjustments frequently result in major gains, so begin implementing these adjustments into your daily schedule and take charge of your PKD journey.

Medications for Blood Pressure Management in Polycystic Kidney Disease

Through my work, I have personally seen the value of an all-encompassing approach to healthcare that incorporates medical interventions with lifestyle changes, self-care practises, and psychological support. By taking a comprehensive strategy, we can effectively address the complex issues associated with Parkinson's disease (PKD) and provide the best possible outcomes for our patients.

Medicines are essential for controlling hypertension in people with PKD. Commonly used pharmaceutical classes include several others, each with unique methods of action and possible side effects. Patients should be fully informed about these drugs, as well as the significance of consistent treatment and routine monitoring.

1. Angiotensin-Converting Enzyme (ACE) Inhibitors:

A class of drugs known as ACE inhibitors functions by preventing the angiotensin-converting enzyme, an enzyme necessary for the synthesis of the hormone angiotensin II, from doing its job. Angiotensin II narrows blood vessels and increases the secretion of aldosterone, a hormone that also causes water and salt retention. ACE inhibitors assist in reducing blood volume and relaxing blood arteries by inhibiting the activity of angiotensin II.

ACE inhibitors such as lisinopril, enalapril, and ramipril are frequently prescribed. Coughing, lightheadedness, dizziness, and a fast heartbeat are possible side effects. When using ACE inhibitors, blood pressure and renal function must be regularly monitored.

2. Angiotensin Receptor Blockers (ARBs):

Angiotensin II receptor antagonists, or ARBs, function by preventing angiotensin II from attaching to its receptors. This results in vasodilation and decreased fluid retention by preventing the hormone from forcing blood vessels to narrow and by reducing the release of aldosterone.

PKD patients frequently use ARBs such as losartan, valsartan, and irbesartan. Fatigue, elevated potassium levels, and lightheadedness are possible side effects. When using ARBs, it's critical to regularly check blood pressure and kidney function.

3. Calcium Channel Blockers:

A class of drugs known as calcium channel blockers prevents calcium from entering blood vessel cells, which causes the blood vessels to relax and blood pressure to drop. The drugs in question fall into two categories: dihydropyridines and non-dihydropyridines.

Amlodipine and nifedipine are examples of dihydropyridine calcium channel blockers, which mainly affect blood vessels and are frequently used as first-line treatment for high blood pressure in Parkinson's disease (PKD). Since they directly affect the heart, non-dihydropyridine calcium channel blockers like verapamil and diltiazem are helpful in treating some cardiac rhythm issues that may be connected to Parkinson's disease (PKD).

Symptoms of calcium channel blockers that are frequently experienced include flushing, disorientation, and ankle swelling. It is imperative to regularly monitor blood pressure and heart rate when using these drugs.

4. Beta Blockers:

The way that beta blockers function is by preventing the release of certain chemicals, such adrenaline, which can raise blood pressure and heart rate. Beta blockers relieve cardiac strain, which lowers blood pressure.

Metoprolol, atenolol, and propranolol are among the beta blockers that are frequently administered. Breathlessness, lightheadedness, and weariness are possible side effects. When using beta blockers, regular blood pressure and heart rate monitoring is crucial.

5. Diuretics:

Diuretics, commonly referred to as water pills, are drugs that aid in decreasing the body's fluid volume and boosting urine production. Both blood volume and blood pressure decline as a result of this. In PKD, diuretics are frequently recommended to treat high blood pressure, especially when fluid retention is a problem.

Diuretics come in several forms, such as potassium-sparing diuretics, thiazide diuretics, and loop diuretics. For PKD, diuretics such as spironolactone, furosemide, and hydrochlorothiazide are frequently recommended. Increased urination, electrolyte imbalances, and low blood pressure are possible side effects. When using diuretics, it is crucial to regularly check blood pressure, renal function, and electrolyte levels.

It is crucial to keep in mind that each person is unique, and the medicine selection may change based on the patient's particular needs and circumstances. It's also important to let your healthcare professional know about all of your drugs and medical problems because some medications may have drug interactions or contraindications.

In order to effectively manage PKD, blood pressure and kidney function must be regularly monitored. This enables medical professionals to evaluate the drugs' efficacy, alter them as needed, and identify any possible negative effects early on. Maintaining ideal blood pressure management and halting additional kidney damage requires strict adherence to treatment, which includes taking prescription drugs as directed and going to check-ups on a regular basis.

In summary, controlling high blood pressure in people with Parkinson's disease (PKD) necessitates a multifaceted strategy that includes drug therapy, lifestyle changes, and routine monitoring. To make educated decisions and take an active role in their own healthcare, people must be aware of the possible side effects and mechanisms of action of the regularly used medications. People with PKD can effectively control their blood pressure, maintain kidney function, and improve their general well-being by collaborating closely with a healthcare team.

Monitoring and Managing Blood Pressure in Polycystic Kidney Disease

In my capacity as a physician and wellness and health coach, I have worked with numerous individuals who have polycystic kidney disease (PKD). Effectively monitoring and controlling blood pressure is one of the most important parts of managing this illness. I will discuss the value of self-monitoring, goal blood pressure ranges, routine blood pressure monitoring, and the need of honest communication with medical experts in the management of Parkinson's disease (PKD) in this subchapter.

Kidney cyst formation is a hallmark of progressive kidney disease (PKD), a chronic and complex kidney disease. Over time, these cysts may progressively become larger, which may cause a number of issues, including elevated blood pressure. As a matter of fact, among the most frequent issues that people with PKD experience is high blood pressure. According to studies, between 50 and 75 percent of persons with PKD experience hypertension by the time they are 60 years old.

Regular monitoring is the first step towards effectively managing blood pressure in people with PKD. People with PKD are advised to regularly check their blood pressure, especially those who are more vulnerable—for example, those with a family history of high blood pressure or impaired kidney function. This makes it possible to identify any variations or anomalies early on and to take swift action to stop any problems.

For people with PKD, target blood pressure ranges can change according on their age, general health, and the existence of additional comorbidities. Nonetheless, as a broad recommendation, the majority of specialists concur that people with PKD should aim for a blood pressure of less than 130/80 mmHg. It is important to remember that these figures could vary based on a person's unique situation.

Consulting with medical professionals is crucial to figuring out what the best goal blood pressure range is for each individual.

For those with PKD, self-monitoring is essential to blood pressure management. People who routinely check their own blood pressure at home can better manage their health and make educated decisions about changing their lifestyle and, if needed, changing their medications. Self-monitoring not only gives people the ability to take control of their health but also makes it possible to comprehend their condition and how it is progressing more thoroughly.

Using a trustworthy and accurate blood pressure monitor is essential for self-monitoring blood pressure at home. The market offers a variety of varieties, from completely automated electronic monitors to manual monitors with stethoscopes. Seeking advice from a healthcare practitioner is recommended when determining which gadget best suits a person's needs and preferences.

To properly manage blood pressure in patients with Parkinson's disease (PKD), open communication with healthcare professionals is crucial in addition to routine monitoring. Frequent examinations and consultations with a medical team that specialises in Parkinson's disease (PKD) can assist in detecting and quickly resolving any emerging or current problems. To guarantee ideal blood pressure control, these experts can offer tailored guidance on food adjustments, lifestyle adjustments, and medication management.

Changes in lifestyle are essential for controlling blood pressure in people with PKD. Regular physical activity can help lower blood pressure and enhance cardiovascular health in general. Examples of this activity include walking, swimming, and cycling. Blood pressure levels can also be significantly impacted by eating a healthy, balanced diet low in processed foods and sodium and high in fruits, vegetables, whole grains, and lean proteins.

For those with PKD, counselling and psychologically based methods can be helpful in controlling blood pressure. Anxiety and stress can raise blood pressure, and chronic illnesses can have a negative impact on mental health. Stress can be reduced and blood pressure can be managed by using stress-reduction strategies like mindfulness, meditation, deep breathing exercises, and engaging in enjoyable and relaxing hobbies and activities.

A thorough blood pressure management plan might include a variety of complementary and alternative self-care strategies. Herbal treatments, acupuncture, and naturopathy are examples of alternative therapies that may be good for blood pressure. Before beginning any complementary or alternative therapy, it is imperative to speak with a healthcare provider because these treatments should be incorporated into the entire treatment plan under the supervision of a qualified healthcare provider.

Additionally essential to overcoming the difficulties of controlling blood pressure in PKD are coping mechanisms. Making the connection with support groups or individual counselling can offer a secure setting for sharing experiences, voicing worries, and learning from others going through comparable struggles. Effective blood pressure management and general well-being can benefit from the emotional support these contacts provide.

To sum up, controlling and monitoring blood pressure on a regular basis is essential for the treatment of polycystic kidney disease. Maintaining blood pressure within desired levels will help stop more issues from arising and enhance general well-being. Effective blood pressure management in Parkinson's disease (PKD) requires self-monitoring, lifestyle adjustments, open communication with healthcare experts, and incorporation of complementary and alternative approaches and coping strategies. People with PKD can empower themselves to take charge of their health and guarantee the best results by managing their blood pressure holistically and proactively.

Chapter 10: Polycystic Kidney Disease and Pregnancy

Fertility and Polycystic Kidney Disease

A delicate and complex component of one's general health is fertility. Kidney cysts can interfere with the reproductive system and make it difficult for PKD patients to become pregnant. It is essential for those who want to start a family or properly manage their reproductive health to understand how PKD impacts fertility.

It is important to understand that both men and women can be impacted by PKD and fertility. Men may experience structural abnormalities in the reproductive organs, such as seminal vesicles or an enlarged or cyst-filled epididymis. Infertility may arise from these anomalies if there is a decrease in sperm count, motility, or even a total lack of sperm.

When it comes to reproduction, women with PKD have particular difficulties. Kidney cysts can cause problems for the reproductive system's regular operation. Women with PKD frequently experience hormonal imbalances, which can interfere with ovulation and the regular menstrual cycle and make conception challenging. Furthermore, PKD-related issues like high blood pressure and renal insufficiency can raise the chance of miscarriage, early delivery, and other pregnancy-related issues.

People with PKD and their spouses should seek appropriate medical therapies and help to manage these issues. Seeking advice from a reproductive endocrinologist or fertility expert who has dealt with renal disease patients in the past can be very beneficial. To maximise the possibilities of conception, these specialists can evaluate the individual reproductive issues and provide customised treatment programmes.

In many cases, treating hormonal imbalances is an essential first step in treating PKD-related infertility problems. For women, hormone therapy may be suggested to control ovulation and encourage regular menstrual periods. In vitro fertilisation (IVF) and intrauterine insemination (IUI) are two assisted reproductive methods that may provide effective treatment for men who are having fertility problems.

For people with PKD, lifestyle changes are crucial in controlling their fertility and reproductive health in addition to pharmacological therapies. It's especially crucial to reach and maintain a healthy weight because obesity can exacerbate hormone imbalances and make fertility issues more difficult. In order to give my patients with individualised food regimens that will support their reproductive health, I frequently work with nutritionists and dieticians.

During this journey, psychological assistance and stress management strategies are especially important because dealing with fertility issues can have an enormous emotional toll. In order to relieve stress and improve their general well-being, I advise my patients to investigate complementary therapies like acupuncture, meditation, and counselling.

Proactively addressing any worries or anxieties regarding PKD and fertility is crucial. Making use of counselling services designed especially for people dealing with PKD and infertility issues or joining support groups can offer a secure setting where people can talk about their experiences, let out their frustrations, and receive emotional support from others who have firsthand knowledge of the difficulties.

Other family-building methods should be taken into consideration if PKD difficulties make conception impossible or too dangerous. For people and couples who have a strong desire for a child, adoption and surrogacy provide alternate routes to parenting that can lead to great happiness and satisfaction.

Undoubtedly, PKD has a significant effect on fertility and reproductive health, but it's important to remember that there are resources and support available to help people deal with these challenges. Resolving infertility issues related to PKD can be greatly increased by consulting a physician, making lifestyle changes, and taking care of one's emotional health.

Recall that you are not travelling alone. You can approach your fertility and reproductive health goals with confidence, resilience, and the knowledge that it might take some time, patience, and adaptability if you have access to the correct resources, support, and information. You are the creator of your own path, and while PKD may cause challenges, it does not limit your capacity to build the family you want.

Pregnancy Planning and Preconception Care for Polycystic Kidney Disease

Genetic counselling is among the most crucial elements of pregnancy preparation for individuals with Parkinson's disease. Since PKD is a hereditary condition, it can be inherited from either or both parents. For those with PKD who intend to become parents, it is essential that they comprehend the hereditary ramifications and the hazards linked to the condition. Patients who receive genetic counselling are given important information regarding the probability of PKD being passed down to their offspring and the potential severity of the disease in subsequent generations. Patients can make well-informed decisions regarding family planning and acquire a thorough understanding of the PKD inheritance pattern through genetic counselling.

Moreover, genetic counselling can assist in determining the presence of any additional genetic abnormalities or illnesses that may coexist with PKD. This is especially crucial because some genetic disorders might make pregnancy much more difficult and necessitate further medical procedures. Patients with Parkinson's disease (PKD) can make sure they have a thorough awareness of their genetic composition by receiving genetic counselling. This will help them make decisions about their reproductive health and the welfare of their offspring down the road.

Another essential part of PKD patients' preconception care is medication management. Working closely with their healthcare team, people with PKD must evaluate the safety and suitability of their existing drugs for use during pregnancy. Certain drugs that are frequently recommended for peripheral kidney disease (PKD), like angiotensin receptor blockers (ARBs) and angiotensin-converting enzyme inhibitors (ACE inhibitors), may be harmful to the growing foetus. To reduce any possible hazards, it is crucial to find substitute medications or change the dosage.

For PKD patients, lifestyle changes are essential for improving pregnancy outcomes in addition to drug management. Throughout pregnancy, leading a healthy lifestyle can have a significant impact on the mother's and the unborn child's general health. Making lifestyle changes is especially more important for those with PKD because it can have a direct effect on how quickly the condition progresses.

First and foremost, it's important to keep your food well-balanced. Patients with PKD should concentrate on eating a low-sodium diet to assist control their blood pressure. It is important to stress the eating of whole foods, such as fruits, vegetables, whole grains, and lean proteins. It's also strongly advised to cut out on processed foods, sugar-filled drinks, and saturated fats. For those with Parkinson's disease (PKD), maintaining adequate hydration is especially crucial since it helps support kidney health and reduce the risk of kidney stones.

Another major lifestyle change that can help people with PKD is regular exercise. Walking, swimming, or cycling are examples of moderate-intensity exercises that can help you maintain a healthy weight and enhance your cardiovascular health in general. Before beginning any workout programme, it's crucial to speak with a healthcare provider to make sure it's safe and suitable for your particular situation.

Techniques for managing stress are also essential for PKD patients' preconception treatment. Prolonged stress can worsen PKD symptoms and have a detrimental effect on general health and wellness. Reducing stress and fostering a sense of peace and relaxation can be achieved by engaging in stress-reduction practises including deep breathing exercises, mindfulness, and meditation. Getting help from a mental health professional or joining PKD-specific support groups can also help in managing the emotional difficulties that are frequently associated with the illness.

Patients with Parkinson's disease (PKD) need to learn coping mechanisms to help them deal with the psychological and physical effects of the illness. Overall wellbeing can be greatly enhanced by partaking in joyful and fulfilling activities, such as hobbies, creative pursuits, or quality time spent with loved ones. Patients with Parkinson's disease (PKD) should also be conscious of their limits and exercise self-care by getting enough sleep when needed and getting support when needed.

In summary, preconception care and pregnancy planning are critical for people with Parkinson's disease. Patients with Parkinson's disease (PKD) can increase their chances of a successful and healthy pregnancy by following lifestyle adjustments, taking appropriate medication, and participating in genetic counselling. Patients must collaborate closely with their medical team to develop a customised plan that takes into account their particular requirements and situation. PKD patients can start their road towards parenting with confidence and peace of mind if they receive the right preconception treatment.

Pregnancy Complications and Management in Polycystic Kidney Disease

For any woman, being pregnant is a joyful and transformative event. Women who have Polycystic Kidney Disease (PKD) may face particular difficulties and worries as a result. As a physician with a focus on holistic medicine and wellness, I have worked with numerous PKD patients who have successfully navigated the pregnancy process. I'll provide you important advice and ideas on managing your PKD while pregnant in this subchapter.

Regular Prenatal Care:

Regular prenatal care is one of the most important parts of managing PKD during pregnancy. A series of appointments with your healthcare practitioner are part of prenatal care. Your healthcare professional will check your general health and well-being as well as do numerous tests throughout these sessions.

These routine examinations are much more important for women who have PKD. Your doctor will check your blood pressure, renal function, and look for any indications of potential problems. They could request urine, blood, and ultrasound tests to evaluate the development and well-being of your child.

Your healthcare practitioner can identify any potential problems early on with regular prenatal care. Many issues can be avoided or successfully controlled with early intervention and appropriate management.

Monitoring Kidney Function:

Throughout your pregnancy, it is crucial to keep a close eye on your kidney function as a patient with PKD. Your kidneys are under more stress during pregnancy, so it's important to make sure they're operating at their best. Your kidney health can be ascertained using routine blood tests, such as those that measure creatinine and estimated glomerular filtration rate (eGFR).

One common consequence in both PKD and pregnancy is high blood pressure. It's critical to maintain your blood pressure if you want to save your kidneys and make sure you and your unborn child are healthy.

Your doctor will keep a careful eye on your blood pressure and might recommend medicine to lower it. It is imperative that you take these drugs as prescribed and that you take your blood pressure at home on a regular basis. Your doctor may change the dosage of your medication or suggest other lifestyle changes if your blood pressure starts to rise.

Management of High Blood Pressure and Other Pregnancy-Related Issues:

Patients with progressive kidney disease (PKD) need to take care of a few additional pregnancy-related concerns in addition to controlling hypertension and keeping an eye on kidney function. You can effectively traverse these challenges if you prepare and arm yourself with the knowledge and tools you need.

Diet and Nutrition:

It's imperative that you keep up a nutritious, well-balanced diet during pregnancy for the health of both you and your unborn child. You should be aware of particular dietary issues as a patient with PKD, such as lowering your sodium consumption to assist control blood pressure.

Seeking advice from a qualified dietician with expertise in renal health can offer you priceless direction and encouragement. They can assist you in creating a customised meal plan that satisfies your dietary requirements and takes into account the particular difficulties associated with prenatal PKD.

Furthermore, maintaining proper hydration is critical for kidney health. It aids in your body's removal of waste materials and pollutants.

Try to stay hydrated by drinking lots of water and consuming as few caffeine-containing beverages as possible.

Exercise and Physical Activity:

Pregnancy-related benefits of regular exercise include increased mental and physical health, less risk of gestational diabetes, and enhanced cardiovascular health. It is imperative, therefore, to speak with your healthcare provider prior to beginning or extending an exercise regimen.

Low-impact activities like swimming, walking, and prenatal yoga can be very helpful for PKD patients. These are low-impact activities that improve cardiovascular health without overtaxing your kidneys and are easy on your joints.

Rest and Stress Management:

Stress management is essential for your general well-being throughout pregnancy because it can be a physically and emotionally taxing time. Deep breathing exercises, meditation, and prenatal massage are examples of relaxation practises that can be incorporated to assist reduce stress and foster a sense of peace and well-being.

During your pregnancy, it's imperative to give rest and good sleep first priority. Pay attention to your body and take pauses when necessary. Resting enough facilitates healing and supports healthy kidney function.

Coping Strategies and Support:

It can be extremely difficult to manage the difficulties of pregnancy while having PKD at times. For your mental and emotional health, you must learn coping mechanisms and get help.

Joining PKD-specific online forums and support groups is something you should think about. Developing a connection with people who have experienced comparable things helps foster understanding and a sense of community. It's also a chance to get advice, information, and emotional support from others who really get your experience.

In conclusion, women with PKD may face particular difficulties during pregnancy. However, you can effectively navigate this path if you plan ahead and take regular prenatal care along with management techniques. Always put your health and wellbeing first, and don't hesitate to ask your healthcare practitioner for advice and assistance when needed. I am here to support you at every stage of your journey into motherhood, which is one to be treasured and enjoyed.

Postpartum Care and Family Planning for Polycystic Kidney Disease

It is critical for PKD patients to concentrate on their postpartum care following childbirth. The physical strain of pregnancy and childbirth takes time for the body to heal. This recuperation is even more important for PKD-afflicted women because their kidneys may have been under more stress during pregnancy.

In my capacity as a physician and health and wellness coach, I emphasise the value of continuing to follow PKD patients after giving birth. It is essential to have regular check-ups with your healthcare practitioner to make sure that there are no pregnancy-related issues and that your kidney function is stable. Blood pressure monitoring, urine testing to look for indications of kidney damage, and imaging procedures such as MRIs or ultrasounds to determine the size and quantity of kidney cysts should all be part of these examinations.

During the postpartum phase, it's equally critical to focus on your general health and wellbeing. This entails leading a healthy lifestyle that includes consistent exercise, a well-balanced diet, and enough sleep. Deep breathing exercises, yoga, meditation, and other stress-reduction and self-care methods can all contribute to general well-being.

It is crucial for PKD patients to think about safe and effective contraceptive methods while planning their families, as long as they don't raise their risk of kidney problems. For women with PKD, hormonal contraceptives—such as birth control pills, patches, or injections—are usually regarded as safe. Talking about this with your healthcare professional is crucial, though, as there might be certain factors to take into account given your unique health situation.

The copper intrauterine device is another reliable and safe method of contraception for people with Parkinson's disease (IUD). A medical professional can implant this non-hormonal method of contraception, which offers long-term protection against unintended births. To be sure this option is right for you, it is crucial to talk about it with your healthcare provider.

Patients with Parkinson's disease (PKD) may occasionally decide to have sterilising operations like vasectomy or tubal ligation. These operations should be carefully evaluated, taking into consideration individual circumstances and personal choices, as they are permanent types of contraception. It's critical to go over the advantages and disadvantages of these treatments in detail with your healthcare professional.

Patients with Parkinson's disease (PKD) should talk to their doctor before thinking about getting pregnant again in order to weigh the risks and make an educated choice. Pregnancy is not prohibited by PKD per se, although the disorder may affect fertility and raise the possibility of pregnancy-related problems including hypertension or preeclampsia.

It is crucial for women with PKD who intend to become pregnant to meet with their healthcare physician for preconception counselling. During this appointment, you will be able to go over any worries or inquiries you may have, assess your general health, and create a customised plan for managing your PKD while pregnant.

Patients with progressive kidney disease (PKD) may need more regular check-ups and closer monitoring throughout pregnancy to maintain stable kidney function and general health. It will be crucial to do routine blood pressure checks and urine testing to look for any indications of kidney impairment or other issues. Your doctor might occasionally advise imaging tests like an MRI or ultrasound to check for kidney cyst growth and track any changes.

Maintaining a healthy lifestyle throughout pregnancy is also essential, emphasising a balanced diet, frequent exercise, and enough sleep. This will reduce the possibility of issues and enhance your general well-being.

In conclusion, PKD patients need to carefully examine and manage their family planning and postpartum care. To make sure that there are no pregnancy-related problems during the postpartum phase, continuous monitoring of kidney function is crucial. It's important to talk about contraception alternatives with medical professionals to make sure they're safe and effective for persons with Parkinson's disease. Preconception counselling and closer monitoring throughout pregnancy are crucial when making plans for future pregnancies in order to reduce risks and guarantee the best possible outcome. PKD patients can confidently manage family planning and postpartum care by following these guidelines and collaborating closely with healthcare professionals. This will enable them to live a happy and healthy life.

Chapter 11: Emotional Support and Mental Well-being in Polycystic Kidney Disease

The Psychological Impact of Polycystic Kidney Disease

People with Parkinson's disease (PKD) frequently experience anxiety, depression, and grief as emotional responses. Patients may experience severe anxiety in response to the surprise of learning they have a chronic condition, which can leave them feeling helpless and apprehensive about the future. A persistent underlying dread can be brought on by ongoing concerns about the course of the disease, the likelihood of requiring kidney transplantation or dialysis, and the potential effects of PKD on their quality of life. As a result, bodily signs of anxiety may include restlessness, trouble sleeping, and even panic attacks.

Another common psychological reaction to PKD is depression. Feelings of despondency and sadness can arise due to the chronic nature of the disease and the possibility of physical discomfort and limits. Patients may suffer changes in appetite or weight, trouble concentrating, an overall lack of desire, and a loss of interest in once-enjoyed activities. The difficulties in treating the illness can be made worse by depression, which has a substantial negative influence on general wellbeing.

Grief is arguably one of the most important psychological effects of Parkinson's disease. A diagnosis of a chronic illness invariably includes a tremendous sense of loss, and grief is a normal reaction to any kind of loss. Patients may experience sadness about losing their prior state of health, their unrestricted ability to participate in particular activities, and their hopes and dreams for the future. As they observe the steady deterioration in their renal health, they could also lament the loss of their kidney function. Grief can elicit a wide range of emotions, including acceptance, sadness, and anger. It is important to negotiate these feelings with consideration and compassion.

It is critical to identify and validate these affective responses in people with Parkinson's disease (PKD) and to offer them support during their journey. It is important to recognise that the psychological effects of Parkinson's disease (PKD) can have a substantial impact on an individual's general well-being and capacity to properly manage their illness. Healthcare providers and loved ones can foster a supportive atmosphere that promotes candid conversation and emotional healing by addressing these feelings.

It's critical to investigate different coping mechanisms that can assist patients with anxiety symptoms feel better. Reducing anxiety and fostering calm can be greatly aided by deep breathing exercises, mindfulness practises, and meditation. Regular physical activity that improves general wellbeing, like yoga or walking, can also help reduce stress and anxiety.

When it comes to depression, a multifaceted strategy is crucial. Patients should be encouraged to undertake self-care behaviours that support emotional well-being in addition to seeking professional assistance from mental health specialists. A balanced diet, consistent exercise, and getting enough sleep are all crucial aspects of self-care that can improve mental and emotional well-being. In addition, participating in therapeutic activities like art therapy or journaling, or asking for support from support groups, can allow people a way to express their feelings and find comfort.

Grief is a complicated feeling that needs room and time to heal. It is important to support patients with PKD in using support groups, group therapy, or individual counselling to work through their feelings of loss. It is critical to provide a secure, encouraging space free from criticism or judgement where patients can express their grief. Healthcare professionals and loved ones can help people navigate the different stages of grieving and find acceptance and serenity by listening with compassion and validating their emotions.

In summary, it is imperative to consider the psychological effects of Parkinson's disease (PKD) when pursuing all-encompassing healthcare and managing the illness. Patients and their loved ones may frequently experience anxiety, sadness, and grief. It is important to provide coping mechanisms, support, and validation to assist people manage these difficult feelings. Healthcare providers and loved ones can improve the general health and quality of life for those with Parkinson's disease (PKD) by creating an atmosphere of empathy and understanding. Keep in mind that you have resources at your disposal to help you throughout the entire road, and you are not alone on this one.

Coping Strategies for Emotional Challenges in Polycystic Kidney Disease

Activities for self-care are crucial for handling emotional difficulties in PKD. Taking care of oneself has many different facets, such as mental, emotional, and physical self-care. Exercise on a regular basis, mindfulness and meditation practises, eating a balanced diet, and getting adequate sleep are all essential aspects of self-care that support emotional health. Endorphins, sometimes referred to as "feel-good" hormones, are released when you exercise and can help reduce tension and anxiety. In a similar vein, engaging in mindfulness and meditation practises can assist people in developing a feeling of peace and relaxation, lessening the effects of emotional difficulties.

For those with PKD, nutrition is essential for coping with emotional difficulties. Eating a healthy, well-balanced diet can assist control mood and general wellbeing. To create a food plan that meets your unique needs, speak with a medical practitioner or a registered dietitian who specialises in Parkinson's disease (PKD). It may be helpful to include foods that are known to improve mood, such as omega-3 fatty acids, which are present in nuts, seeds, and fish. Emotional well-being can also be improved by consuming fewer processed and sugary meals and drinking enough of water.

In addition to proper diet and physical self-care, finding joy in life and fulfilling activities is crucial for overcoming emotional obstacles. Passions, interests, and hobbies can be constructive diversionaries and means of self-expression. Spending time on hobbies that bring you joy, such as painting, music making, gardening, or any other pastime, can reduce stress and enhance your mental health in general. Participating in activities that provide a feeling of success and purpose might be especially beneficial for people with Parkinson's disease (PKD), as they may encounter constraints as a result of their illness.

Creating a network of support is another essential step in managing emotional difficulties in Parkinson's disease. Being in the company of perceptive and sympathetic people can give one a feeling of community, lessen feelings of loneliness, and provide much-needed emotional support. Support groups designed especially for people with PKD can be very helpful since they offer a forum for people to share experiences, exchange knowledge, and find comfort in the company of others who genuinely comprehend the difficulties related to the condition. Support groups provide a forum for people to exchange thoughts, learn from each other's coping mechanisms, and rediscover hope.

Counseling and therapy can be very helpful in addressing emotional difficulties associated with Parkinson's disease. Getting professional assistance from a therapist or counsellor with expertise in mental health and chronic illness can offer people a secure and encouraging setting in which to examine and manage their feelings. Therapy can assist people in overcoming the challenges of living with Parkinson's disease (PKD), addressing underlying psychological disorders, and developing useful coping methods. One treatment strategy that is frequently used to help people with chronic illnesses manage their emotional well-being is cognitive-behavioral therapy (CBT). CBT focuses on recognising and refuting unfavourable ideas and attitudes in order to encourage more positive emotional reactions.

Alternative and complementary therapies can be investigated as coping mechanisms for emotional difficulties in Parkinson's disease (PKD) in addition to conventional therapy. Acupuncture, yoga, massage therapy, and aromatherapy are among the techniques that have demonstrated encouraging outcomes in enhancing emotional well-being, lowering tension and anxiety, and encouraging relaxation. To ensure safety and efficacy, it is crucial to get advice from medical professionals before implementing these approaches into a coping strategy.

A customised strategy is necessary to develop appropriate coping techniques for emotional problems in Parkinson's disease (PKD) because every person's experience with the condition is different. While controlling emotions can be difficult and may take some time and practise, it is important to be patient and kind to oneself during the coping process. For a thorough and all-encompassing approach to addressing emotional issues in Parkinson's disease (PKD), consulting with a multidisciplinary team of healthcare specialists, psychologists, nutritionists, and practitioners of alternative therapies can be beneficial.

Through self-care practises, networking, therapy, counselling, and investigating complementary and alternative methods, people with PKD can create a toolkit of coping mechanisms that support mental health. It takes a lifetime to manage emotional difficulties, but with the correct tools and assistance, people with PKD can thrive in spite of their illness and manage the difficulties of daily life. Recall that you are not travelling alone on this road, and that by advancing your emotional health, you are giving yourself the ability to live a happy and purposeful life.

Seeking Professional Help for Mental Health in Polycystic Kidney Disease

It can be an emotionally taxing experience to live with PKD. Anxiety, despair, and extreme stress might result from the many doctor's appointments, the unknown future, and the possible effects on day-to-day living. Given the profound effects that these mental health issues can have on an individual's general wellbeing, it is imperative that they be recognised and addressed.

Psychologists are experts in mental health who focus on comprehending human behaviour, ideas, and emotions as well as the underlying reasons of these phenomena. They can be extremely helpful in assisting people with PKD in managing the emotional difficulties that come with the illness. Psychologists can assist patients in processing their feelings, creating useful coping mechanisms, and enhancing their general mental health by offering treatment and counselling.

It is essential to locate a psychologist with experience treating chronic illnesses such as PKD when seeking professional help for mental health issues related to the disease. These psychologists can offer specialised help and guidance because they are aware of the particular difficulties faced by people with long-term illnesses. They can support patients in overcoming PKD's emotional ups and downs and building resilience in the face of hardship.

Another helpful option for those with PKD who are looking for professional assistance for mental health issues is counsellors. Counselors, as opposed to psychologists, usually concentrate more on advice and support than on therapy. They can support patients in discovering their strengths, exploring their feelings, and creating mental health management plans.

Psychologists and counsellors frequently collaborate, sending patients to each other when therapy is required. They can also provide advice on how to handle stress, practise self-care, and make lifestyle changes that will improve mental health. Counselors can help patients with PKD navigate the emotional difficulties brought on by the condition and help them maintain a healthy, balanced lifestyle in spite of it.

People with PKD may occasionally need more comprehensive mental health care, which may include medication management. Herein lies the role of psychiatrists. Licensed medical professionals with a focus on mental health and the ability to prescribe medicines are known as psychiatrists. They are able to determine if medication is necessary and track how well it works to address mental health issues associated with Parkinson's disease.

Finding a psychiatrist who is knowledgeable about mental health disorders and the consequences of PKD is crucial when seeking professional care for mental health in the disease. This knowledge guarantees that patients receive all-encompassing care that considers their mental health requirements as well as the possible effects of Parkinson's disease on their general health.

Psychiatrists can administer medicine and offer counselling services. For those with more serious mental health issues, this medicine plus therapy combo can be quite helpful. It makes it possible to treat the illness holistically, taking care of its biological and psychological components.

It is crucial to understand that getting professional assistance for mental health issues among people with PKD does not indicate weakness or a lack of coping skills. Rather, it is an indication of resilience and self-awareness. Being aware of when one needs more help and actively seeking it out shows that one is committed to their own mental health.

Better coping mechanisms, increased emotional resilience, and an all-around higher quality of life can result from doing this. People with PKD can better manage the disease's effects on their daily life by attending to mental health issues, which promotes a sense of empowerment and control.

In summary, getting professional assistance for mental health issues in people with Parkinson's disease is crucial to providing holistic treatment. When needed, psychiatrists, psychologists, and counsellors can offer helpful advice, treatment, and medication management. They can assist those who have Parkinson's disease (PKD) in managing the emotional effects of the illness, creating useful coping mechanisms, and enhancing their general mental health.

It's critical to locate experts who have worked with people who suffer from chronic illnesses such as PKD. These experts can offer PKD patients specialised help and guidance because they are aware of the particular difficulties they confront.

Recall that asking for assistance is a sign of strength rather than weakness. You are investing in your general well-being and strengthening your capacity to deal with any obstacles that post-ketonergic diarrhoea may bring. Accept the help at your disposal and give yourself the tools you need to lead a happy life despite having PKD.

Building a Support Network in Polycystic Kidney Disease

Managing Polycystic Kidney Disease (PKD) can be an isolating and daunting experience at times. I have direct experience as a physician and health and wellness coach with the positive effects that a robust support system may have on the quality of life for people with Parkinson's disease (PKD). The purpose of this subchapter is to provide light on the significance of creating such a network and how it can support both disease management and general well-being.

It's important to first define a support network's scope in order to fully appreciate its relevance. A support network in the context of Parkinson's disease disease (PKD) is a collection of individuals who offer the patient practical, emotional, and physical support. Other PKD patients, as well as family, friends, and medical professionals, can be a part of this network. Each of these people has a special role to play in the patient's journey, providing information, support, and empathy to help the patient deal with the difficulties associated with Parkinson's disease.

The opportunity to exchange experiences and gain knowledge from one another is among the most beneficial elements of interacting with other PKD sufferers. The knowledge that they are not alone in their troubles can be comforting for patients through support groups, internet forums, or in-person meetups. They can feel more connected to others and have their own feelings validated by hearing about others' experiences with comparable difficulties. Patients can also learn about different therapy options, coping mechanisms, and lifestyle changes that have been successful for other people. Patients who are empowered to actively participate in their own health and treatment strategies might benefit from this shared information.

Although establishing connections with other individuals with Parkinson's disease (PKD) is crucial, family support is an invaluable resource. For people with PKD, family members frequently act as their primary caregivers and emotional supports. They give unwavering love and support as they see the everyday setbacks and victories. In order to improve understanding and communication between the patient and their loved ones, it is imperative to nurture these ties. In addition to fostering closer ties among family members, talking about worries, anxieties, and hopes lessens the stress of dealing with the illness.

Friends can also be an important part of a patient's network of support for Parkinson's disease. These people provide an alternative viewpoint and frequently act as a diversion and a return to normalcy. A quick phone call, coffee date, or movie night with friends can offer much-needed relief from the medical requirements of Parkinson's disease. Friends help patients' mental and general well-being by providing a brief distraction from their concerns.

The medical community, which consists of physicians, nurses, and therapists, is equally crucial to the support system. These people can offer priceless advice and medical expertise because they have specific understanding and experience managing Parkinson's disease (PKD). Building strong bonds with medical staff guarantees that patients get the finest treatment and information available. This partnership makes it possible to manage diseases with a more all-encompassing strategy that addresses psychological and emotional as well as physical factors.

Knowing oneself and one's needs and preferences is the first step in establishing and maintaining helpful partnerships. While some people might do better in big support groups, others might prefer one-on-one conversations. It's critical to investigate several options and determine which ones are most effective for each patient. Patients with Parkinson's disease can connect with others who are going through similar experiences through social media groups, online forums, and local support groups. Seeking out expert resources can also offer a secure setting for talking about emotional difficulties and creating coping mechanisms. Examples of these professionals include therapists and counsellors who specialise in chronic disease.

Establishing a network of support calls for efforts and active involvement. Patients ought to initiate social interactions, go to support group gatherings, and participate in conversations. However, setting limits and giving self-care first priority are as crucial. Taking on too much at once might result in burnout and increased stress. Maintaining general well-being requires making time for self-care and recharging.

In summary, creating a support system is essential to controlling polycystic kidney disease. Developing relationships with other patients, family members, friends, and medical professionals has several advantages, such as knowledge exchange, emotional support, and helpful guidance. Patients with Parkinson's disease (PKD) can discover comfort, strength, and hope again by cultivating these relationships. Recall that you are not travelling alone, and that by working together, we can overcome the difficulties presented by PKD.

Chapter 12: Polycystic Kidney Disease and Children

Polycystic Kidney Disease in Infants and Young Children

In my capacity as a doctor who specialises in holistic medicine and wellbeing, I have treated many patients with polycystic kidney disease (PKD), including young children and newborns. Even though adult patients are frequently linked to PKD, it's crucial to understand that people with this genetic illness can also be affected from a very young age. Indeed, research has demonstrated that PKD can appear in foetuses as early as the prenatal stage.

The absence of overt symptoms in the early stages of PKD in newborns and young children presents a diagnostic problem. Pregnancy-related routine ultrasounds frequently reveal the presence of PKD. When kidney cysts are detected by these ultrasounds, more testing may be necessary to confirm the diagnosis. It is crucial to remember that not all PKD instances are identified during pregnancy, and some newborns may exhibit symptoms later in life.

PKD symptoms in newborns and early children might change based on how severe the condition is. Physical examination can determine the presence of enlarged kidneys in neonates in certain instances. On the other hand, if the cysts enlarge over time, they may put strain on surrounding tissues and organs, which could result in consequences. Urinary tract infections, excessive blood pressure, and even renal failure are examples of these consequences. Since effective management of PKD depends on early intervention, it is imperative to keep an eye out for any indicators of severe issues in newborns and early children.

Infants and young children with PKD may have growth abnormalities and developmental delays in addition to physical symptoms. This is because the kidneys' dysfunction has an effect on how the body functions as a whole. The synthesis of hormones that are necessary for growth and development is just one of the many biological processes that the kidneys regulate with such precision. Developmental delays and restricted growth may occur when kidney function is compromised by cystic growth. As a result, it's critical that paediatric doctors keep a close eye on the development and growth of kids with PKD and offer the right interventions to promote their general wellbeing.

For PKD to be effectively managed in newborns and early childhood, early diagnosis is essential. Early diagnosis of Parkinson's disease (PKD) allows medical professionals to create a thorough care plan that minimises the disease's negative effects on the child's health. This plan can involve doing imaging studies to track the development of cysts, regular blood testing to evaluate kidney function, and adopting lifestyle changes to support kidney health.

Pediatricians are essential in the treatment of PKD in newborns and early children. These healthcare providers can offer solutions that are specifically designed to address the requirements of young patients since they have received specialised training and skill in paediatric care. Particularly paediatric nephrologists are qualified to handle the intricacies of PKD in this age range. They can offer advice on how to take medications, change one's diet, and keep an eye out for any possible problems. Furthermore, they work closely with other professionals, such dietitians and psychiatrists, to guarantee a comprehensive approach to treatment.

A comprehensive approach is necessary for the therapy of paediatric patients with PKD. Treating the child's and their family's emotional and psychological needs is equally as important as treating the physical symptoms. PKD is a chronic illness that can be difficult to manage, especially for young children and their parents. Therefore, in order to assist children and their families in navigating the complexity of the disease, it is crucial that healthcare providers provide counselling and support services. To help families dealing with comparable issues, this may entail establishing peer support groups, offering resources for emotional support, and teaching coping mechanisms.

In summary, PKD can affect newborns and early children, necessitating an early diagnosis and all-encompassing treatment plans. To give these young patients the best care possible, it is crucial to understand the probable indications and symptoms of this ailment as well as the role paediatric doctors play in managing it. Children with Parkinson's disease (PKD) can have happy, productive lives and successfully manage their condition if their medical care is provided in a holistic manner that addresses both the physical and emotional components of the illness.

Polycystic Kidney Disease in School-Age Children and Adolescents

School-age children and adolescents may experience notable growth and developmental delays as a result of polycystic kidney disease. Kidney function may be impacted by the enlargement of the kidneys brought on by the formation of kidney cysts. Reduced kidney function and poor blood waste product filtering may follow from this. Children who have reduced kidney function may exhibit symptoms like lethargy, disorientation, and appetite loss. High blood pressure, recurrent UTIs, and discomfort in the abdomen can also result from enlarged kidneys. The ability of a child to flourish academically, socially, and emotionally can be significantly impacted by these symptoms.

When managing Parkinson's disease (PKD) in children and adolescents of school age, routine monitoring is crucial. This entails routine check-ups with the doctor for physical examinations, blood tests to evaluate kidney function, and imaging investigations to track the development of cysts and the disease's course. Monitoring makes it possible to identify issues early on and aids in the creation of a treatment plan that is suitable for the child. Additionally, it helps medical professionals to spot any possible roadblocks to efficient care, such prescription non-compliance or lifestyle changes.

In order to effectively manage PKD in school-age children and adolescents, age-appropriate lifestyle adjustments are essential. These adjustments could involve exercising, changing one's nutrition, and learning stress-reduction strategies. A balanced, kidney-friendly diet is crucial for children with Parkinson's disease (PKD) management. This involves reducing the amount of protein consumed to lessen the strain on the kidneys, lowering the amount of salt consumed to regulate blood pressure, and promoting the consumption of fruits and vegetables to supply vital nutrients. Personalized meal plans that consider the child's age, nutritional requirements, and tastes can be created by a qualified nutritionist.

In addition to being good for general health, exercise can aid school-age children and adolescents with PKD. Frequent exercise helps build muscles, lower blood pressure, and enhance general wellbeing. It is imperative to select exercises that are safe and do not overburden the kidneys. Youngsters of all fitness levels can enjoy well-tolerated activities including walking, cycling, and swimming. Getting kids involved in sports or other enjoyable extracurricular activities can also improve their social skills and sense of self.

Another crucial component of PKD management in children and adolescents of school age is stress management. Children may find the diagnosis and treatment of a chronic illness to be emotionally taxing, so it's important to provide them the support and coping mechanisms they need. Children can benefit from counselling and psychology-related practises like cognitive-behavioral therapy to learn appropriate coping mechanisms for stress and to address any emotional issues they may be having. It's crucial to promote open communication and give kids a secure environment in which to voice their worries and feelings.

Self-care practises and coping mechanisms, in addition to alterations in lifestyle, can be quite helpful in the management of PKD in school-age children and adolescents. Children can feel more empowered and in charge of their health when they are encouraged to actively participate in their own care. Acquiring self-help skills like mindfulness, deep breathing exercises, and relaxation techniques will assist individuals in managing any discomfort they may have, be it physical or emotional. Emphasizing the value of self-care and giving kids the resources they require to effectively advocate for themselves and manage their conditions are crucial.

In conclusion, a thorough and all-encompassing approach is needed to address PKD in school-age children and adolescents.

Regular monitoring and intervention are necessary to optimise kidney function and general health due to the possible impact on growth and development. Age-appropriate lifestyle adjustments, such as dietary adjustments, physical activity, and stress reduction methods, are essential to the disease's management. Even with the difficulties presented by PKD, we can help children live happy, healthy lives by using these tactics and giving them self-care and coping mechanisms.

Support and Resources for Parents and Caregivers of Children With Polycystic Kidney Disease

For both the child and the parents, receiving a polycystic kidney disease (PKD) diagnosis can be a daunting experience. Adapting to the diagnosis and treating the illness calls for a comprehensive strategy that includes not just medical attention but also psychological assistance and resource access.

I am committed to offering families impacted by Parkinson's disease (PKD) thorough help in my capacity as a medical practitioner and health and fitness coach. In my practise, I collaborate with a group of specialists from many wellness and health domains to give parents and caregivers the instruments and resources they require to effectively manage this complicated illness.

Education is the first step in helping parents and other caregivers. Families must be fully informed about the nature of paediatric kidney disease (PKD), how it impacts the kidneys, and what the long-term prognosis may be. By arming parents with current and accurate information about Parkinson's disease (PKD), they may make well-informed decisions regarding their child's medical care and guarantee the best possible care.

For parents and other caregivers of children with PKD, advocacy is equally essential. It entails actively searching for skilled medical professionals with PKD management experience and speaking out for their child's particular requirements. This can entail locating paediatric nephrologists and renal dietitians who are skilled in treating children with PKD and can offer individualised therapy. It is imperative that parents take the initiative to speak up for their child's medical needs and make sure they get the finest care available.

Another essential component of caring for kids with PKD is emotional support. Parents and caregivers should have a support structure in place since the strain and unpredictability of treating a chronic condition can be taxing. Making connections with other families experiencing comparable circumstances can bring much-needed understanding and empathy. Online and in-person support groups can provide a secure environment where parents can express their worries, pose inquiries, and find comfort in their shared experience.

For children with PKD, finding expert healthcare practitioners is essential to the overall management of the condition. Physicians who specialise in the diagnosis and treatment of kidney problems in children are known as paediatric nephrologists. They are qualified to handle the special difficulties that kids with PKD encounter and are able to offer all-encompassing treatment. Renal dietitians play a crucial role in ensuring that kids with PKD eat a balanced, healthful diet that promotes the function of their kidneys.

Families impacted by PKD can get information and help from foundations and organisations in addition to medical professionals. These clubs frequently provide parents and caregivers with educational resources, internet discussion boards, and support groups. They can be a very helpful source of knowledge, direction, and emotional support.

The PKD Foundation is one such group that works to advance PKD research, education, advocacy, and support for PKD patients and their families. They provide an abundance of resources, such as webinars, educational materials, and a nationwide network of support groups. In order to provide families with hope for the future, the PKD Foundation also finances research into developing improved treatments and a cure for PKD.

The Polycystic Kidney Disease Foundation (PKDF), which offers assistance and resources to families impacted by PKD, is another important resource. They include informational materials, a resource directory to assist families in locating qualified healthcare providers, and a helpline manned by qualified individuals who may offer advice and answers to queries. The PKDF also plans conferences and events so that families can meet and share the most recent findings in medical research and treatment alternatives.

Apart from these organisations, parents and caregivers can also establish connections with each other through social media groups and online forums. These groups offer a forum for exchanging insights, posing queries, and locating assistance. Knowing that you are not travelling alone and that there are people who can relate to your struggles and provide support and guidance can be reassuring.

Being a physician and a health and wellness coach, I am committed to helping parents and other caregivers manage Parkinson's disease in their kids. Through knowledge, advocacy, and emotional support, my goal is to enable families to better manage the intricacies of this condition. I firmly think that parents and other caregivers can become true champions for their child's health and wellbeing if they are given the proper guidance and tools.

In summary, in order to ensure the best potential results for children with PKD, it is imperative to provide support to their parents and caregivers. In this process, education, advocacy, and emotional support are essential and can assist parents in taking charge of their child's care. Through establishing connections with PKD-focused groups and specialist healthcare practitioners, parents and caregivers can obtain the necessary resources to effectively manage this intricate condition. Recall that you are not alone on this path and that you can give your child with PKD the finest care possible if you have the correct assistance.

Transitioning to Adult Care in Polycystic Kidney Disease

Making the switch from childhood to adult care is a big step for people with polycystic kidney disease (PKD). It signifies the entry into maturity and has its own unique set of difficulties and factors to take into account. As a physician and health and wellness coach, I have personally observed the challenges that patients have during this time of change. I hope to give my patients the knowledge and resources they need to effectively traverse this phase by offering a thorough guidance on the transition to adult care in PKD in this section.

For many PKD patients, the switch from paediatric to adult care can be a difficult one. It entails a number of adjustments, such as switching to a new healthcare team or provider, taking on the responsibility of maintaining one's health on one's own, and adjusting to the disparities between the healthcare systems for adults and children. Additionally, because of the abrupt change in responsibilities and the unknowns that lie ahead, young adults with PKD may experience psychological and emotional difficulties throughout this transition.

During this moment of transformation, continuous monitoring is one of the most important factors to take into account. Since PKD is a chronic illness that needs to be managed over time, it's essential to see medical professionals on a regular basis to avoid complications and guarantee the best possible results. On the other hand, paediatric and adult treatment may use different monitoring strategies. While patient autonomy and self-management are more important in adult care, disease control and parental involvement are frequently the main points of attention in paediatric care.

Healthcare providers must offer education and assistance that is specifically designed to meet the requirements of young adults with

Parkinson's disease (PKD) in order to facilitate a seamless transition. This entails providing patients with the information and abilities they need to successfully manage their illness, such as self-care practises, lifestyle adjustments, and medication management. Involving the patient in decision-making processes is crucial because it fosters their autonomy and gives them the power to actively participate in their medical care.

The assistance that healthcare professionals provide during the transition to adult care is another important factor to consider. I support a holistic approach to healthcare and wellness as a medical doctor and health and wellness coach. Therefore, I serve PKD patients during this transitional period by assembling a multidisciplinary team of experts from several sectors related to health and wellness.

For instance, patients may profit from the knowledge of nutritionists, who may design a diet specifically tailored to each patient's needs and health objectives. A nutritionist's advice can be very helpful in helping young individuals make educated decisions and build healthy eating habits, as diet is a key component of controlling Parkinson's disease (PKD). Furthermore, mental health specialists like psychologists or counsellors can help patients manage the psychological and emotional components of the shift and help them overcome any obstacles they may face.

Additionally, any other comorbidities or lifestyle issues that can affect the general health and well-being of individuals with Parkinson's disease (PKD) should be addressed throughout the transition phase. Young adults with PKD, for example, might be more likely to get cardiovascular disease or hypertension. Thus, working together with cardiologists and other medical specialists can guarantee thorough treatment and efficient management of these ailments.

In summary, the move from paediatric to adult care in PKD is an important stage in the patients' life. It necessitates carefully weighing the difficulties and factors particular to this transitional phase. A smooth transition process requires constant observation, patient education, and the assistance of a multidisciplinary team. In my capacity as a physician and wellness and health coach, I'm dedicated to giving my patients the resources and encouragement they need to get through this stage confidently and reach their best health possible. I will go into more detail about particular methods and approaches in the upcoming chapters, which can facilitate PKD patients' successful transition to adult care.

Chapter 13: Polycystic Kidney Disease Research and Future Directions

Current Research in Polycystic Kidney Disease

Being up to date on medical research is essential to me as a medical practitioner and health and wellness coach. It enables me to give my patients with Polycystic Kidney Disease (PKD), a difficult and complex illness that affects millions of people globally, the best care possible. Thanks to the diligent efforts of researchers worldwide, our understanding of Parkinson's disease (PKD) has significantly advanced in recent years. I will explore some of the most important discoveries made in the field of PKD research to date in this subchapter, along with the exciting new directions that these studies have opened up for possible treatment approaches.

Investigating possible therapeutic targets is one of the most fascinating parts of modern PKD research. Numerous cellular and molecular pathways have been found to be essential to the onset and course of Parkinson's disease (PKD). We can create tailored treatments that directly target the disease's fundamental causes by comprehending these pathways.

For instance, it has been found that one of the main factors for cyst growth in PKD is deregulation of the cyclic adenosine monophosphate (cAMP) pathway. Potential PKD therapies include drugs that can return this route to its normal functioning. Moreover, recent research has demonstrated that PKD cyst formation can be slowed down by inhibiting a protein known as mammalian target of rapamycin, or mTOR. PKD patients are presently undergoing clinical trials to assess mTOR inhibitors' effectiveness in treating the condition.

PKD is mostly influenced by genetics, and scientists have made great strides in figuring out which genes cause the illness. The most prevalent type of PKD, autosomal dominant PKD (ADPKD), is brought on by mutations in either the PKD1 or PKD2 gene. Through examining these genes, scientists intend to improve their comprehension of the mechanisms underlying the disease and create specialised treatments.

The development of next-generation sequencing methods has significantly advanced genetic research on Parkinson's disease (PKD) in recent years. Using these methods, scientists can examine a patient's whole genome to find new genetic variations linked to Parkinson's disease (PKD). This information has improved our comprehension of the genetic causes of Parkinson's disease (PKD) and created new avenues for individualised treatment.

Another area of active PKD research is biomarkers. Measurable components in the body known as biomarkers can reveal details about the course of a disease, how it responds to therapy, and its overall prognosis. Finding trustworthy PKD biomarkers is essential for early diagnosis, tracking the course of the illness, and evaluating the effectiveness of treatment.

Recent years have seen the identification of a number of putative biomarkers, such as those related to kidney function, fibrosis, and inflammation. For instance, research has demonstrated that increased levels of specific cytokines, such as TNF-alpha (TNF-alpha) and interleukin-6 (IL-6), are linked to deteriorating kidney function and faster cyst formation in individuals with progressive kidney disease (PKD). By keeping an eye on these indicators, we can learn a great deal about how diseases develop and adjust our treatment strategies accordingly.

Our capacity to thoroughly research PKD has also been transformed by sophisticated imaging methods. We can see cysts and follow their development over time with high-resolution pictures of the kidneys obtained from computed tomography (CT) and magnetic resonance imaging (MRI). Furthermore, novel imaging techniques like diffusion-weighted MRI have demonstrated potential in identifying fibrosis early in Parkinson's disease.

Through the integration of these sophisticated imaging techniques with biomarker studies, scientists want to create non-invasive approaches for tracking the advancement of diseases and evaluating the effectiveness of treatments. By removing the need for invasive treatments like kidney biopsies and offering a more complete view of the disease, this would significantly improve patient care.

In summary, present PKD research endeavours are yielding noteworthy advancements in augmenting our comprehension of the ailment and crafting focused treatments. The future of PKD management is quite promising as long as possible targets for treatment are identified, the genetic basis of PKD is investigated, and biomarkers are found. I'm eager to apply these developments to my work as a physician and health and wellness coach so that I can give my patients the best, most individualised care possible. Keeping up with the most recent research results allows me to continue providing my patients with the information and resources they need to live happy, meaningful lives despite the difficulties posed by Parkinson's disease.

Emerging Treatment Options for Polycystic Kidney Disease

The complicated genetic disease known as PKD is typified by the development of many kidney cysts. Gradually growing cysts have the potential to cause kidney enlargement, loss in renal function, and ultimately kidney failure. For many years, the main goals of PKD treatment have been to reduce symptoms and delay the course of the illness. But new findings have raised hopes for ground-breaking therapies that might slow the progression of this illness.

This subchapter will discuss novel surgical approaches, gene treatments, and possible pharmaceutical interventions that may be able to reduce the course of PKD and improve patient outcomes.

Pharmacological Interventions:

One crucial component of treating Parkinson's disease is the use of pharmaceuticals. Certain elements of the disease, such as cyst formation, inflammation, and deterioration in kidney function, are targeted by these treatments. While most modern drugs concentrate mostly on treating symptoms, novel therapies try to address the underlying causes of Parkinson's disease and stop the disease's progression.

The creation of pharmaceutical medicines that specifically target the growth of cysts is one noteworthy field of research. Numerous biochemical targets and pathways, including the cyclic adenosine monophosphate (cAMP) and mammalian target of rapamycin (mTOR) pathways, have been found to be involved in the creation and growth of cysts by researchers. The goal of focusing on these pathways is to prevent the creation of cysts and possibly halt the course of the disease.

Early-stage clinical studies and promising preclinical research have demonstrated that some drugs, such tolvaptan, may be able to delay the progression of Parkinson's disease. In patients with Parkinson's disease (PKD), tolvaptan, a selective vasopressin V2 receptor antagonist, has shown promise in reducing kidney enlargement and maintaining renal function. To ascertain the medication's safety and long-term effects, more research is being conducted.

Gene Therapies:

Research on gene treatments has shown promise in treating Parkinson's disease (PKD). PKD is a hereditary condition that arises from mutations in particular genes, including PKD1 and PKD2. The goal of gene treatments is to compensate for these genetic defects in order to return kidney function to normal.

One method of gene therapy is the use of gene silencing tools, including short interfering RNA (siRNA). Genes that cause disease can be specifically targeted by siRNA molecules to inhibit their expression. Researchers have focused on PKD1 gene expression in the context of PKD to prevent cyst development and expansion.

These gene-silencing treatments have produced encouraging outcomes in animal models of Parkinson's disease, while being in the experimental stage. They have successfully slowed the formation of cysts and enhanced renal function. In order to evaluate the safety and effectiveness of these treatments in people, more investigation and clinical testing will be required in the future.

Innovative Surgical Techniques:

Historically, surgical treatments have only been used to treat PKD-related problems like bleeding or infected cysts. Recent developments in surgical methods, however, present fresh options for the treatment of PKD.

Laparoscopic cyst decortication is one such procedure that includes removing the cyst lining while leaving the healthy kidney tissue intact. In certain individuals with large or symptomatic cysts, this technique has demonstrated promise in lowering pain, enhancing kidney function, and delaying the course of the disease.

The transplantation of bioengineered kidneys is another cutting-edge surgical technique. Researchers are investigating the use of donor kidneys that have been decellularized—that is, stripped of all cellular components—as a scaffold for the growth of new kidneys derived from patients' own stem cells. By substituting healthy, working kidneys for the damaged ones, this ground-breaking method may provide those with PKD a new lease on life.

Even if these new therapy alternatives have a lot of promise, we should approach them cautiously optimistically. Thorough investigation, lengthy clinical testing, and regulatory clearances are required to guarantee their efficacy and safety. It's also critical to keep in mind that managing Parkinson's disease (PKD) is complex and calls for an all-encompassing strategy that include self-care practises, food planning, counselling, and lifestyle alterations.

In conclusion, new and innovative treatment options for people with PKD are constantly being developed by the field of study in this area. There is promise for bettering outcomes and decreasing the progression of disease thanks to developments in gene treatments, pharmaceutical interventions, and surgical methods. I'm determined to keep you updated and give you the support you need to properly handle PKD as we continue to understand its complexity. By working together, we can overcome the difficulties caused by PKD and pursue ideal health and well-being.

Patient Involvement in Polycystic Kidney Disease Research

Clinical trials are essential to the advancement of medicine and the enhancement of patient outcomes. They are crucial to the creation of fresh PKD medicines and treatments. Patients who take part in clinical trials may have access to innovative therapies that aren't readily available elsewhere. Patients who volunteer for a clinical trial take an active role in their own healthcare and open the door for future patients to profit from the research.

Enrolling in a clinical study has advantages that go beyond the personal gains of the participant. Patients can influence future treatment options and raise the standard of care by adding to the corpus of knowledge about Parkinson's disease (PKD). Patients and their families can feel empowered and filled with optimism as a result of this involvement. They might find comfort in the knowledge that their involvement can significantly improve the lives of those who are impacted by this illness.

However, what about patient databases? What impact do they have on PKD research? Databases that gather and preserve data on people identified as having a specific ailment are called patient registries. These registries offer researchers useful information that they can use to assess treatment outcomes, find patterns, and get a deeper understanding of the condition. Patients with Parkinson's disease (PKD) can make sure that their experiences and medical history are recorded by actively participating in patient registries. This will help to create a greater body of knowledge that will ultimately inform future research and development.

Another essential component of patient involvement is pushing for research funding and awareness, in addition to taking part in clinical studies and patient registries. Because PKD is a complicated and multidimensional illness, more study is needed to solve its riddles and develop more potent cures. Patients and their families can help spread the word about PKD and gain support from legislators, researchers, and the general public by speaking out in favour of the condition. This enhanced awareness may result in more money and resources being allocated to PKD research, which would speed up the creation of new therapies and enhance patient outcomes.

There are many different ways to be an advocate, from telling your own storey and having conversations with elected leaders to organising fundraisers. Patients who want to connect with others going through similar struggles and work together to achieve a common goal can also join patient support groups or charitable organisations devoted to Parkinson's disease. Patients have the ability to influence significant change and propel PKD research forward when they band together and raise their voices.

Recognizing that patient participation in research is a two-way street is crucial. Throughout the study process, scientists and medical practitioners should actively seek out and value patient input. Researchers can make sure that their study is truly patient-centered and meets the most urgent needs of the PKD community by using patient perspectives, concerns, and priorities. More significant and lasting outcomes may arise from patient participation in study design, data analysis, and findings distribution.

As a physician and health and wellness coach, I am a firm believer in the benefits of holistic healthcare, which takes into account a patient's emotional and psychological requirements in addition to their physical health. Living with Parkinson's disease (PKD) can be an arduous and physically and mentally taxing experience. To improve their quality of life, I thus advise patients to experiment with different self-care complementary and alternative treatments, self-help tactics, and coping mechanisms.

To assist patients in managing the psychological and emotional aspects of living with Parkinson's disease (PKD), a variety of methods are available, ranging from mindfulness meditation and relaxation techniques to dietary adjustments and stress management tactics. These methods can provide a comprehensive approach to managing Parkinson's disease (PKD) and enable individuals to take charge of their own health and well-being when paired with medical treatments and therapies.

To sum up, patient participation in PKD research is critical to the advancement of medical knowledge, the enhancement of therapy options, and the improvement of patient outcomes. Patients may improve the lives of persons with PKD and pave the way for future breakthroughs by taking part in clinical trials and patient registries, which will add to the body of knowledge around the condition. In addition, it is essential to promote research funding and awareness in order to advance the field and guarantee that the needs of the PKD community come first. We can make PKD patients' futures more promising by actively incorporating them in research and offering them comprehensive care.

Future Directions in Polycystic Kidney Disease Research

The future of PKD research appears to be brightly promising in the field of precision medicine. The goal of precision medicine is to customise medical care for each patient by taking into account their distinctive genetic composition, environment, and lifestyle choices. PKD is a complicated illness that varies from person to person in terms of severity and course. By allowing medical professionals to create tailored treatments based on the unique features of each patient's condition, precision medicine has the potential to completely transform the management of Parkinson's disease.

Genomic medicine is one field of precision medicine that has great promise for PKD research. After it was finished in 2003, the Human Genome Project gave scientists a plethora of knowledge about the human genome and how diseases arise. Researchers can find genetic variants and mutations linked to PKD by sequencing the genomes of patients. Personalized treatments that target these particular genetic anomalies can then be created using the information provided, thereby delaying the progression of the disease and improving patient outcomes.

Furthermore, new avenues for treating Parkinson's disease (PKD) at its source are made possible by technological advancements like CRISPR-Cas9 and other gene editing approaches. With the use of CRISPR-Cas9, scientists may precisely alter the DNA sequence to fix genetic abnormalities that result in illnesses like Parkinson's disease. Gene editing is a rapidly developing topic with tremendous potential for treating Parkinson's disease (PKD), even if it is still in its early phases of development.

Additionally, personalised treatments have a lot of potential for treating Parkinson's disease. Although there is presently no known cure for PKD, patients' quality of life can be increased, symptoms can be reduced, and the disease's course can be slowed down with individualised treatment plans. Healthcare professionals can create individualised treatment regimens that are particular to each patient by considering criteria such as age, gender, lifestyle choices, and the severity of the illness.

Targeted pharmacological therapies are one area of tailored medicine that is gaining popularity in PKD research. Using drugs or other treatments that particularly target the mechanisms behind the onset and progression of Parkinson's disease (PKD) is known as targeted therapy. For instance, new research indicates that certain medications, including tolvaptan, can inhibit the development of kidney cysts in people with Parkinson's disease. The discovery of additional medications that can specifically target certain PKD pathways may result in the creation of more potent therapeutic alternatives.

Furthermore, the development of artificial intelligence (AI) has the potential to completely change how PKD is diagnosed and treated. Massive volumes of medical data, such as genetic data, imaging investigations, and patient histories, can be analysed by AI algorithms to find trends and generate precise forecasts regarding the course of a disease and its response to treatment. Healthcare professionals may make better decisions and offer individualised advice for each patient by utilising AI.

Early disease detection is one area in which AI can significantly advance PKD research. At the moment, PKD is frequently misdiagnosed until severe symptoms appear and irreversible kidney damage has taken place. AI systems are able to examine patient data and spot trends that point to the existence of Parkinson's disease (PKD), enabling early diagnosis and therapy. Prompt identification has the ability to avert or postpone the necessity for dialysis or transplantation, as well as greatly enhance patient outcomes.

AI can also help in the creation of predictive models that evaluate PKD patients' likelihood of illness progression. Artificial intelligence (AI) systems can produce individualised risk scores that predict the likelihood of illness development and complications by evaluating genetic and clinical data. Healthcare professionals can use this information to create more individualised treatment programmes and to decide whether to do procedures like transplants.

In summary, the field of PKD research has a bright future ahead of it thanks to developments in personalised medicine, artificial intelligence, and precision medicine. These research fields have promising opportunities to enhance PKD patients' diagnosis and treatment results. I'm committed to remaining on top of these developments as a medical professional and health and wellness coach so that I can give my patients the finest care possible. By combining these cutting-edge strategies with PKD care, we can create a thorough plan for managing polycystic kidney disease that takes into consideration the unique requirements and traits of every patient.

Chapter 14: Polycystic Kidney Disease and Other Health Conditions

Hypertension and Polycystic Kidney Disease

Subchapter 1: The Relationship between Hypertension and PKD

As a physician and health and wellness coach, I find that hypertension, or high blood pressure, is one of the most prevalent illnesses among my patients with polycystic kidney disease (PKD). There is no denying the link between these two illnesses, and people with PKD need to be aware of how hypertension may affect their kidney function. This subchapter will examine the connection between PKD and hypertension, outlining the possible effects of high blood pressure on kidney health and stressing the significance of blood pressure control for the successful management of both disorders.

It is predicted that 60–70% of people with PKD will experience hypertension at some point in their lives. The strong association between these two situations is demonstrated by this statistic. Comprehending the variables that contribute to this correlation can assist us in formulating efficacious tactics for concurrently managing them.

One of the hallmarks of Parkinson's disease (PKD) is the development of kidney cysts, which can cause a number of issues, including hypertension. The kidneys get larger and lose their natural structure and function as a result of the cysts in PKD gradually getting bigger over time. The complex interplay of hormones and other components involved in blood pressure regulation is upset by this structural change.

The renin-angiotensin-aldosterone system is one of the main pathways that connect hypertension with Parkinson's disease (RAAS). Cyst enlargement throws off the delicate balance between the parts of this system in people with Parkinson's disease (PKD), which results in an atypically active RAAS. Due to this activation, angiotensin II levels rise, which is a strong vasoconstrictor that raises blood pressure. Consequently, hypertension emerges as a common characteristic among PKD patients.

Subchapter 2: The Impact of High Blood Pressure on Kidney Function

Now that we know the connection between PKD and hypertension, let's examine the possible effects of high blood pressure on kidney health. Uncontrolled hypertension can worsen the damage done to the kidneys by making PKD worse and hastening the development of renal failure.

The blood arteries in the kidneys are under more stress when blood pressure is up. Nephrosclerosis is a disorder that develops when the arteries are harmed over time by this continuous pressure. The term "nephrosclerosis" describes the hardening and scarring of the renal blood vessels, which reduces the kidneys' capacity to receive oxygen and nutrients. Kidney function deteriorates as a result, and cyst formation could worsen.

Furthermore, an excess of protein in the urine, known as albuminuria, might be facilitated by hypertension. A reduction in renal function is indicated by the presence of albuminuria, a sign of kidney disease. When high blood pressure and albuminuria are present in people with PKD, the kidney disease advances more quickly, endangering the patient's general health.

Subchapter 3: The Importance of Blood Pressure Control

It is crucial to stress the importance of blood pressure regulation because of the significant effects that high blood pressure can have on kidney function and PKD. In addition to lowering the risk of cardiovascular problems, controlling hypertension effectively is also essential for maintaining renal health and delaying the onset of Parkinson's disease.

The American Heart Association recommends that the target blood pressure for those with PKD be less than 130/80 mmHg.

Reaching this objective can be difficult, especially in light of the difficulties in concurrently controlling PKD and hypertension. As a result, a comprehensive strategy that includes medication, lifestyle changes, and routine monitoring is crucial.

I frequently collaborate extensively with my patients to create all-encompassing medication regimens for the management of their PKD and hypertension. Changes in lifestyle are essential for controlling blood pressure. These include eating a heart-healthy diet, getting regular exercise, controlling stress, abstaining from tobacco and excessive alcohol use, and managing stress. Furthermore, controlling weight is essential because even a small reduction in weight can have a big effect on blood pressure.

In many cases, medication is required to get the desired blood pressure values. People with PKD are frequently taken ACE inhibitors and angiotensin receptor blockers (ARBs), which have been demonstrated to reduce the growth of kidney cysts in addition to helping manage blood pressure. But it's crucial to remember that medicine should always be administered by a doctor and closely watched over.

Subchapter 4: Challenges in Managing Hypertension and PKD

For some people, managing PKD and hypertension at the same time can be difficult. There is a risk that illness management will lapse due to the complexity of medication schedules, lifestyle changes, and routine monitoring. It is essential to address the difficulties patients encounter and give them the resources and assistance they need to successfully complete this trip.

Medication adherence is a common difficulty in the management of PKD and hypertension. For some people, taking many drugs and following a strict schedule can be challenging, especially if they struggle with side effects or forgetting to take their pills. In my role as a health and wellness coach, I frequently collaborate directly with patients to create plans for enhancing medication adherence, including reminding people to take their medications, utilising pill organisers, and educating them on the value of doing so.

The change of lifestyle patterns presents another difficulty. It takes effort and dedication to adopt a heart-healthy diet, incorporate regular exercise, and manage stress. Making these changes might be difficult for many people, so it's important to give them resources and continuous assistance. Collaborating with a group of specialists that includes dietitians, fitness instructors, and mental health counsellors can improve the efficacy of lifestyle changes and promote long-term success.

A comprehensive strategy that takes into account the mental, emotional, and physical components of both disorders is needed to manage PKD and hypertension at the same time. Counseling and psychology-related approaches are essential in assisting people in managing their stress, creating coping mechanisms, and overcoming the emotional difficulties brought on by chronic illnesses. Incorporating complementary and alternative therapies, like yoga, meditation, and acupuncture, can also improve general wellbeing and offer extra support.

In summary, there is a complex and significant link between PKD and hypertension. People who have kidney disease (PKD) should be aware of the substantial impact that high blood pressure can have on kidney function and general health. Through lifestyle improvements, blood pressure control, and addressing the difficulties associated with treating both disorders at the same time, people can take charge of their health and slow the progression of Parkinson's disease. By adopting a holistic strategy that integrates multiple healthcare domains and tactics, we can enable people with Parkinson's disease to fully experience life and achieve optimal health and wellness.

Diabetes and Polycystic Kidney Disease

Despite being two very different medical illnesses, diabetes and polycystic kidney disease (PKD) frequently coexist, posing a complex combination of issues for patients. I have treated many patients with both diabetes and Parkinson's disease (PKD) in my capacity as a physician and health and wellness coach. It's critical to comprehend how these disorders interact with one another and how renal function may be affected.

Initially, diabetes—especially type 2 diabetes—may be harmful to the kidneys. Damage to the kidneys' small blood capillaries may result from persistently high blood sugar levels. The disease known as diabetic nephropathy can develop as a result of this damage over time, which can impede the kidneys' capacity to remove waste from the circulation. The coexistence of diabetes and PKD may worsen the problem because kidney cysts can obstruct regular kidney function, making it more difficult for the kidneys to efficiently filter waste.

Furthermore, elevated blood pressure can result from both diabetes and PKD, which exacerbates kidney injury. The confluence of these ailments may result in a vicious cycle in which declining kidney function raises blood pressure, which then exacerbates the kidney damage.

Patients have a distinct set of difficulties when managing both diabetes and Parkinson's disease. Blood sugar regulation is one of the main priorities in this regard. Maintaining steady blood sugar levels is essential for diabetics in order to stop further kidney damage. This means using insulin or oral hypoglycemic medicines as directed by a doctor, monitoring blood glucose levels on a regular basis, and embracing a healthy lifestyle that includes regular exercise and a balanced diet.

However, when PKD is involved, blood sugar management may become more difficult. It may be more difficult to attain stable blood sugar control when PKD is present because it can alter how the body reacts to insulin. Higher blood sugar levels may result from kidney cysts that obstruct the absorption of insulin as they expand. This calls for a customised approach to managing diabetes, maybe involving medication adjustments and regular monitoring to guarantee ideal blood sugar control.

Kidney damage prevention is another important part of controlling these illnesses. Blood pressure management is crucial for maintaining kidney function in diabetics. If blood pressure falls outside of a healthy range, medication may be recommended to control it. In addition, blood pressure can be effectively controlled by a low-sodium diet, frequent exercise, and stress reduction methods. Moreover, people with PKD need to avoid variables that could hasten the development of cysts and kidney damage, as well as be aware of how their kidneys work.

A patient's mental health may be significantly impacted by managing both diabetes and Parkinson's disease (PKD) at the same time. Stress, worry, and even melancholy may grow because to the hassle of keeping an eye on blood sugar levels, following intricate drug schedules, and even dealing with renal problems. In addition to giving patients coping mechanisms, counselling, and support, it is imperative to treat these psychological components.

I understand the value of treating the full patient—not just their medical issues—as a physician who supports holistic healthcare and wellness. I stress the value of self-care practises and stress management in addition to advocating lifestyle changes like a balanced diet and consistent exercise. Stress reduction and general well-being have been demonstrated to be enhanced by methods including deep breathing exercises, yoga, and meditation.

To conclude, there are several facets and a complex association between diabetes and Parkinson's disease. Controlling blood sugar and keeping blood pressure within normal ranges are crucial since both disorders may negatively affect kidney function. Managing both illnesses at the same time is difficult and calls for a customised strategy that fits the unique requirements of each patient. Moreover, a key element of comprehensive care is attending to the psychological aspects and offering patients support. People with PKD and diabetes can take charge of their health and improve their quality of life if we embrace a holistic approach to healthcare.

Liver Disease and Polycystic Kidney Disease

Let us establish these words before we go into the details of liver illness and how it is related to PKD. A genetic condition known as polycystic kidney disease is typified by the development of many kidney cysts. These cysts are fluid-filled sacs that come in different sizes and numbers. Eventually, they cause the kidney to expand and lose some of its functionality. On the other hand, a wide range of illnesses that impact the structure or function of the liver are included in the term "liver disease," including cirrhosis, fatty liver disease, and hepatitis.

Up to 85% of PKD patients will at some point in their lives have liver cysts, which are a typical PKD presentation. The biliary or bile ducts in the liver are usually the source of these cysts. Even though liver cysts by themselves might not show any symptoms, their existence can make PKD issues worse.

Determining the effect of liver cysts on kidney function is one of the major issues in addressing both liver disease and Parkinson's disease. Liver cysts may put strain on the kidneys and other nearby organs, thereby compromising their ability to function. This may cause renal function to deteriorate and cause PKD to proceed more quickly. Additionally, structural alterations in the liver brought on by liver cysts might result in hepatic problems that worsen kidney impairment.

Monitoring on a regular basis is essential for managing PKD and liver disease. This entails regular blood tests to evaluate kidney and liver function as well as imaging tests including CT and ultrasound scans to track the quantity and size of kidney and liver cysts. Healthcare providers can detect any changes or difficulties early on and adjust treatment approaches by constantly monitoring these data.

Lifestyle changes are essential for controlling PKD and liver disease in addition to monitoring. It's crucial to maintain a healthy weight through balanced diet and consistent exercise. Reducing alcohol intake is crucial for people with liver disease since too much of it can exacerbate liver damage. In a similar vein, people with PKD should make an effort to keep their diets low in salt because too much of it might exacerbate renal function by causing fluid retention.

The psychological and emotional effects of having both PKD and liver illness must also be addressed. One's mental health may suffer when dealing with the weight of a chronic illness, therefore it's critical to develop coping mechanisms and get help. I work closely with patients as a health and wellness coach, offering them psychological tools and counselling to help them improve their mental health and overall quality of life.

Potential drug interactions between the drugs used to treat PKD and liver disease should also be taken into account while managing both illnesses concurrently. In order to prevent negative interactions or further harm from occurring from different medications, patients and their healthcare providers must collaborate closely. This can necessitate using different medications that are less likely to cause problems or carefully titrating amounts. Keeping the lines of communication open with medical professionals is crucial to ensuring a thorough and all-encompassing approach to therapy.

In summary, there are many different facets and a complex link between PKD and liver disease. Liver cysts can have a negative impact on renal function, making PKD issues worse. The key to managing two illnesses concurrently is regular monitoring, lifestyle changes, psychological support, and knowledge of pharmaceutical interactions. Together, patients and medical practitioners can traverse the intricacies of PKD and liver disease by thoroughly addressing these factors, which will eventually improve quality of life and health outcomes.

Mental Health Conditions and Polycystic Kidney Disease

It can be difficult to manage polycystic kidney disease (PKD) both physically and psychologically. Mental health may suffer as a result of ongoing concern about the disease's course, multiple doctor visits, and the effect on day-to-day functioning. Studies have revealed that, in comparison to the general population, those with PKD are more prone to suffer from mental health issues such anxiety and depression. Their general well-being and quality of life may be greatly impacted by these mental health issues.

A prevalent mental health issue among people with Parkinson's disease is anxiety. Anxiety levels can rise as a result of the disease's ongoing uncertainty and fear. Ideas like "What if my kidneys fail?" or "Will I need a transplant?" might take up mental space and result in persistent anxiety and fear. Anxiety can also cause physical symptoms like breathing difficulties, a fast heartbeat, and trouble falling asleep. To effectively manage anxiety, it is critical to identify these signs and get the right support.

Another mental health issue that frequently coexists with Parkinson's disease is depression. Feelings of hopelessness, worthlessness, and depression can be exacerbated by the chronic nature of Parkinson's disease (PKD), its effects on physical health, and the lifestyle restrictions that go along with it. The loss of their prior degree of physical health and independence can be difficult for people with Parkinson's disease (PKD), which can cause sadness and sorrow. It is vital to recognise these feelings and get assistance in order to stop depression's detrimental effects on general wellbeing.

It can be especially difficult when PKD and mental health issues coexist. Anxiety and depressive symptoms can make PKD physical symptoms worse, creating a vicious circle of poor health. Anxiety, for instance, can raise stress and blood pressure levels, which may exacerbate renal symptoms and function. However, depression can also deplete one's energy and motivation, making it more difficult to manage the illness with appropriate self-care and lifestyle changes.

PKD management necessitates a comprehensive strategy that takes into account both the psychological and physical aspects of the illness. It is essential that you seek the right help along your path. It is advised to speak with a medical expert, such as a psychologist or psychiatrist, who specialises in both PKD and mental health. They can offer the direction and care required to properly manage mental health disorders, including counselling, medication, or a mix of the two.

To enhance mental health, people with PKD can use a variety of self-help methods in addition to expert assistance. These methods include mindfulness exercises, relaxation techniques, and stress management tactics. Regular physical activity has been shown to improve mental and physical health as well. Exercise can help reduce the symptoms of anxiety and sadness because it releases endorphins, which are naturally occurring mood enhancers.

Coping mechanisms are essential for treating PKD and mental health issues. People can better manage the difficulties of having a chronic illness by learning effective coping strategies. Finding and applying the coping mechanisms that are most effective for each individual is crucial. These could be taking up joyful and fulfilling hobbies or pursuits, keeping up a solid support system of family and friends, and participating in self-compassion and encouraging self-talk.

It is impossible to overstate the influence that mental health issues have on general wellbeing. People with Parkinson's disease (PKD) must put their mental health first and get the help they need. In order to achieve a holistic approach to managing Parkinson's disease (PKD), mental health disorders must be addressed in addition to medical therapies and lifestyle modifications. People with PKD can improve their quality of life and ability to manage the difficulties associated with having a chronic illness by fostering their physical and mental well-being.

In conclusion, polycystic kidney disease and mental health issues including anxiety and depression frequently coexist. These illnesses have a major effect on one's general health and quality of life. In order to manage mental health in addition to Parkinson's disease (PKD), it is critical to identify the signs of anxiety and despair, get the right assistance, and use holistic practises. People with Parkinson's disease (PKD) can improve their quality of life and deal with the difficulties of having a chronic illness by treating both the physical and emotional components of their condition.

Chapter 15: Polycystic Kidney Disease and Aging

Aging and Polycystic Kidney Disease

Our bodies experience a variety of physiological changes as we age. The kidneys are not immune to these changes that occur in our body. It is even more important to comprehend the effects of ageing on kidney function and modify our care approach for patients with polycystic kidney disease (PKD).

We must first examine the morphological and functional alterations that the kidneys undergo as we age in order to fully understand how ageing affects PKD. The function of our kidneys is essential in eliminating surplus fluid and waste materials from our blood. But as time goes on, this filtration method's effectiveness tends to deteriorate. After the age of 40, the kidneys' ability to filter waste products is measured by the glomerular filtration rate (GFR), which falls by about 1 mL/min/year. The loss of nephrons, the kidneys' functional units, as well as modifications to blood vessel health and hormone balance, may be the cause of this slow decline.

For people with Parkinson's disease (PKD), becoming older may make these problems worse. Renal cysts can cause gradual swelling of the kidneys over time, which can interfere with normal kidney function. Cysts can replace healthy renal tissue as they enlarge and proliferate, affecting kidney function and interfering with the filtering process. The long-term health and well-being of people with PKD can be greatly impacted by the confluence of cyst formation and the age-related deterioration in kidney function.

For those with Parkinson's disease (PKD), routine monitoring is crucial, particularly as they get older. Kidney function must be closely monitored in order to spot any deterioration or difficulties early on. Imaging techniques like CT or ultrasound scans can give important information on the growth of cysts and the general health of the kidneys, in addition to the standard blood tests used to evaluate kidney function. Regular monitoring of cyst growth and kidney function allows patients and healthcare practitioners to make well-informed decisions regarding management and treatment strategies.

As people with PKD age, it's critical that they make treatment and lifestyle adjustments that are age-appropriate. Although there isn't a treatment for Parkinson's disease (PKD), several lifestyle changes can help the condition grow more slowly and improve general health. Kidney function and general well-being can be greatly impacted by regular exercise, a healthy weight, and a diet rich in nutrients and well-balanced. For those with Parkinson's disease (PKD), low-impact workouts like swimming or cycling can be especially helpful because they reduce the risk of damage and strain on the kidneys.

As people with Parkinson's disease age, therapeutic alterations may also be required in addition to lifestyle adaptations. It might be necessary to reevaluate or adjust medications that were successful in reducing blood pressure or treating other symptoms early in the course of the illness. Certain drugs may require dosage adjustments when renal function falls in order to avoid problems or unfavourable side effects.

It is noteworthy that every person's experience with Parkinson's disease (PKD) is distinct, and the influence of ageing on the illness can differ. To guarantee the most suitable and individualised management approach, patients and healthcare providers must collaborate and communicate on a regular basis. We can overcome the difficulties brought on by ageing and the complications of PKD together.

In conclusion, polycystic kidney disease (PKD) is greatly impacted by ageing and needs to be carefully managed. Renal function naturally deteriorates with age, and those with PKD may have further difficulties as a result of cyst formation and expansion. It's essential to regularly monitor cyst growth and renal function in order to spot any changes or issues early on. Age-appropriate lifestyle choices, such as regular exercise, a healthy diet, and weight control, can help prevent disease and improve general health. As people with Parkinson's disease mature, treatment modifications might also be required. For people with Parkinson's disease (PKD), we can aim for improved outcomes and a higher quality of life by modifying our management tactics to take the effects of ageing into consideration. So let's set out on this adventure together, well informed of the effects of ageing on Parkinson's disease.

Managing Comorbidities in Older Adults With Polycystic Kidney Disease

Subchapter: Challenges of Managing Multiple Health Conditions

Our bodies go through a lot of changes as we age, making us more vulnerable to certain illnesses. The management of various comorbidities is typically necessary for older persons with Polycystic Kidney Disease (PKD), who also have renal disease. We shall examine these people's difficulties in this chapter and talk about management techniques.

1. Interactions between treatments

Treatment recommendations for additional medical illnesses may occasionally interact with one another when an older adult with PKD is diagnosed with those conditions. Medical practitioners may find this challenging since they must carefully evaluate any possible drug-drug interactions and modify treatment strategies as necessary. For instance, several drugs used to treat hypertension may have negative effects on the kidneys, which may be especially dangerous for those who have peripheral kidney disease (PKD). Conversely, pharmaceuticals administered to treat comorbidities may interact with prescriptions used to alleviate PKD-related symptoms, such as painkillers.

As a holistic healthcare provider, my colleagues and I make sure that every prescription our patients take is carefully examined to reduce the possibility of drug interactions. We collaborate closely with pharmacists and other experts to create individualised treatment programmes that are tailored to each patient's specific requirements. This strategy not only lowers the likelihood of unfavourable occurrences but also encourages improved overall PKD and comorbidity management.

2. Comprehensive geriatric assessments

As PKD frequently manifests in older persons with complex medical demands, full geriatric examinations are essential. These evaluations consider the individual's functional, psychological, and social state in addition to their medical history. Through a comprehensive assessment of the person, we can more effectively recognise and manage any problems that can result from co-occurring conditions.

We take into account the patient's mobility, social support, nutritional status, and cognitive performance during a thorough geriatric examination. We also assess their capacity to oversee self-care activities including nutrition and medication compliance. This all-encompassing method aids in the creation of a complete treatment strategy that considers the particular difficulties older persons with PKD and comorbidities confront.

3. Multidisciplinary care

A team of healthcare specialists from different disciplines must work together to manage complex health issues in older persons. We have formed a multidisciplinary team at my clinic that includes physicians, pharmacists, dietitians, psychologists, and physical therapists. Because each team member contributes their area of expertise, we are able to offer patients complete care that takes into account all facets of their well-being.

We are able to provide tailored treatment plans that include coping mechanisms, food and diet planning, counselling and psychology-related techniques, self-care alternatives and complementary treatments, self-help tactics, and lifestyle modifications thanks to interdisciplinary care. This all-encompassing strategy improves overall health outcomes by assisting older persons with PKD in better managing their comorbidities and renal status.

In addition, our team works together and communicates on a regular basis to guarantee smooth care coordination. By doing so, therapy gaps and overlaps are avoided, resulting in the best possible management of PKD and co-occurring conditions. We place a high priority on routine follow-up visits, which enable us to assess patient progress, modify treatment plans as needed, and quickly address any new issues that may arise.

4. Monitoring and preventive care

In order to effectively manage comorbidities in older persons with PKD, routine monitoring and preventative care are essential. We stress the significance of routine health examinations, screening exams, and immunizations in order to identify any possible issues early on. By being proactive, we can lower the chance of illness development or exacerbation and act quickly to intervene.

We also put a lot of effort into encouraging wholesome lifestyle choices that can postpone or prevent the onset of comorbidities. This entails promoting frequent exercise, keeping up a healthy, balanced diet, controlling stress, and getting enough sleep. We develop a feeling of control and encourage improved general well-being in our patients by giving them the tools they need to actively manage their own health.

In summary, managing comorbidities in older persons with Parkinson's disease (PKD) poses distinct problems that need for an integrated, multidisciplinary strategy. We can offer efficient management techniques by taking into account possible interactions between medicines, doing thorough geriatric assessments, and adopting multidisciplinary care. Preventive care and routine monitoring are essential cornerstones in averting problems and advancing general health. Older persons with Parkinson's disease (PKD) can retain a higher quality of life and attain better health outcomes with a comprehensive strategy.

Maintaining Quality of Life in Older Adults With Polycystic Kidney Disease

Building a solid support network is essential to guaranteeing older persons with Parkinson's disease (PKD) a great quality of life. When it comes to managing the mental and physical toll that comes with having a chronic illness, social support is essential. When it comes to Parkinson's disease (PKD), having a strong support system can assist older persons deal with the ups and downs of the illness, offer companionship, and provide emotional comfort. Encouraging patients to connect with their loved ones, join support groups, or seek professional assistance from a therapist or counsellor when necessary is crucial.

In order to preserve their quality of life, older persons with PKD should also give top priority to advanced care planning. Advanced care planning is making decisions regarding medical treatment ahead of time, particularly in case the patient loses their ability to do so. It's critical to have discussions regarding end-of-life choices, including those pertaining to resuscitation, life-sustaining therapies, and hospice and palliative care. These conversations can promote a person's sense of control and peace of mind by reducing anxiety and ensuring that their wishes are honoured.

Encouraging a high quality of life for older persons with Parkinson's disease (PKD) also requires them to maintain their independence and feeling of purpose. It is normal to consider one's life's purpose as we become older and deal with the difficulties that come with deteriorating physical capabilities. Seniors can preserve their mental and emotional health by taking part in enjoyable and fulfilling activities. It can give patients a sense of purpose and improve their general quality of life to encourage them to take up new interests, volunteer, or pursue creative endeavours. Furthermore, promoting independence in older persons can help them keep up their daily activities and sense of autonomy. This can be achieved by making adjustments to living arrangements and using assistive equipment as needed.

Let's now examine each of these points in more detail and look at certain tactics to help older persons with PKD preserve their quality of life:

1. Social Support:

a. Encourage patients to be open and honest about their wants and worries, as well as to talk to their loved ones about their illness.

b. Encourage them to attend PKD-specific support groups so they can interact with people who are aware of their struggles.

c. Give patients access to online forums and groups where they can interact, exchange tales, and seek guidance.

d. Provide resources for counselling or individual treatment to assist patients in coping with the psychological effects of their illness.

2. Advanced Care Planning:

a. Start a discussion regarding the patient's end-of-life desires, being careful to take into account their objectives and values.

b. Assist senior citizens in completing advance directives to make sure their desires are understood and honoured, such as living wills and healthcare proxies.

c. To make sure their healthcare decisions are in line with their values, patients should be urged to include close friends or family members in the conversation.

d. Give people access to local services, such hospice and palliative care programmes, so they can make educated decisions about their future medical treatment.

3. Maintaining a Sense of Purpose and Independence:

Examine the patient's passions, interests, and pastimes to find strategies to modify these pursuits to fit their present level of ability.

b. Promote mentorship and volunteer programmes that help senior citizens achieve fulfilment and give back to their communities.

c. Talk about how important it is to modify the home, like adding ramps or handrails, to encourage independence and reduce the risk of falls.

d. Disseminate information about mobility scooters and walking aids, two assistive technology that can improve mobility while maintaining autonomy.

In summary, older persons with Parkinson's disease (PKD) have complex needs that necessitate addressing multiple facets of their overall health in order to maintain a high quality of life. People with Parkinson's disease (PKD) can successfully manage the difficulties of ageing and chronic illness management by cultivating social support, participating in advanced care planning, and encouraging a feeling of purpose and independence. In order to help older persons with PKD and their healthcare professionals pursue a meaningful and full life, it is my goal that the advice offered in this subchapter will prove to be a useful tool.

Palliative Care and End-of-Life Considerations in Polycystic Kidney Disease

Regardless of the patient's disease stage, palliative care is a comprehensive approach to care that strives to improve quality of life for those with serious diseases. It is sometimes misinterpreted as end-of-life care. It provides assistance to the patient and their family members by attending to their physical, emotional, psychological, and spiritual needs. We can make sure that patients receive the greatest treatment and support possible throughout their journey by including palliative care into the management of Parkinson's disease.

For patients with Parkinson's disease, palliative care must include effective symptom management. Patients may have a variety of symptoms as the illness worsens, such as pain, exhaustion, nausea, and sleep difficulties. Palliative care employs a multidisciplinary approach with the goal of reducing these symptoms. The use of pharmaceuticals, physical therapy, relaxation methods, and complementary therapies like massage or acupuncture may all be part of this. We can greatly raise the patient's quality of life and general well-being by controlling their symptoms well.

Emotional and mental support is a crucial component of palliative care. Living with Parkinson's disease (PKD) can be difficult and emotionally taxing, and sufferers may feel depressed, anxious, or afraid. Through psychological approaches and counselling, we can assist patients in managing these feelings and creating coping mechanisms. Furthermore, community services and support groups can foster a feeling of community and camaraderie by enabling patients to talk about their experiences and gain knowledge from others going through comparable struggles.

For individuals with Parkinson's disease and their families, making end-of-life decisions and establishing advance directives are crucial decisions. Advance directives are formal legal agreements that enable people to specify their preferences for medical treatment and last wishes in the event that they are unable to communicate or make decisions for themselves. Instructions about resuscitation preferences, life-sustaining care, and organ donation may be included in these documents. Patients can make sure that their desires are honoured and that their loved ones are relieved of the stress of making tough decisions at an already trying time by talking about and recording these preferences in advance.

In PKD, end-of-life care necessitates thoughtful preparation and sympathetic assistance. Patients may have to decide whether to switch to hospice care if their condition worsens. Individuals with life-limiting conditions can get specialised medical and emotional assistance through hospice care. It is centred on managing symptoms and pain, providing emotional and spiritual support, and making sure that dying quietly and respectfully. We can guarantee that people with Parkinson's disease (PKD) receive the best care possible during this delicate period by offering assistance on how to obtain hospice services and coordinating care between healthcare providers.

Palliative care acknowledges the significance of spiritual and existential factors in end-of-life care in addition to medical treatment. Every person's path is different, and how they view death and dying will depend on their philosophical and spiritual views. We can offer a holistic care plan that takes into account the patient's physical, emotional, psychological, and spiritual requirements by recognising and honouring their beliefs.

It is crucial to emphasise that palliative care is not just for people with advanced Parkinson's disease. It can be included right from the start of the treatment plan, offering continuous assistance and guaranteeing that patients get the greatest care possible for the duration of their trip. Palliative care can be provided using proactive measures to improve the patient's quality of life, reduce suffering, and promote overall wellbeing.

In summary, end-of-life issues and palliative care are crucial components of the comprehensive therapy of polycystic kidney disease. We can successfully control symptoms, enhance quality of life, and offer PKD patients and their families comprehensive support by incorporating palliative care into the care plan. We've covered the function of palliative care in symptom management and enhancing quality of life in this chapter, along with some advice on advance directives and end-of-life decision-making. We can make sure that individuals with Parkinson's disease (PKD) receive the kind and comprehensive treatment they need by taking these crucial factors into account.

Chapter 16: Polycystic Kidney Disease and Kidney Transplantation

Indications for Kidney Transplantation in Polycystic Kidney Disease

There are several therapy options available for the management of polycystic kidney disease (PKD). Nevertheless, in certain individuals, the illness may ultimately result in end-stage renal disease (ESRD), a condition in which the kidneys are unable to function normally. Kidney transplantation becomes an option in such instances.

When a patient with PKD reaches the end stage renal disease (ESRD), kidney transplantation gives hope and the possibility of a better quality of life. It offers the chance to swap out damaged kidneys for healthy kidneys from donors, regaining renal function and enhancing general health.

Transplant Eligibility for PKD:

Although kidney transplantation appears to be the best option for people with progressive kidney disease (PKD), not everyone is a good candidate. To be eligible for transplantation, a person must fulfil certain requirements.

The existence of end-stage renal disease is the first need (ESRD). Patients must have renal function deterioration recorded to the point that life support requires a transplant. The standard method for quantifying this reduction is to estimate the glomerular filtration rate (eGFR), a measure of renal function. Transplantation is considered when the eGFR drops below a threshold, usually less than 20 mL/min/ 1.73 m^2.

The lack of surgical and immunosuppressive drug contraindications is a crucial requirement for transplant eligibility. Patients must be in good enough physical health to undertake and recuperate from major surgery like transplantation. People must also be able to endure long-term immunosuppressive treatment, which is necessary to avoid the transplanted kidney being rejected.

Transplant Evaluation and Preparation:

Patients must go through a comprehensive screening to determine whether they are a good candidate for kidney transplantation before the process can begin. A multidisciplinary team of medical experts, including nephrologists, transplant surgeons, coordinators of transplants, and other specialists, usually participate in this review.

An exhaustive medical history and physical examination are the first steps in the evaluation procedure. This aids in the detection of any prospective illnesses that can compromise transplantation outcomes or raise the dangers of immunosuppression and surgery. In addition, imaging exams, laboratory testing, and other diagnostic procedures are carried out in order to evaluate the patient's general health and ascertain the degree of renal dysfunction.

An integral component of the pre-transplant evaluation is the psychological assessment. This facilitates the identification of any psychological problems that can affect a patient's capacity to handle the demands of transplantation and the care that follows. Additionally, it gives patients a chance to talk about their thoughts, worries, and expectations around the transplant procedure.

Surgery preparation starts as soon as the patient is judged suitable for transplantation once the examination is finished. This entails taking care of any underlying medical issues, enhancing general health, and making sure the patient is psychologically and emotionally ready for the transplant procedure.

The Potential Benefits of Kidney Transplantation:

A kidney transplant may be beneficial for people with PKD in a number of ways. First and foremost, it offers the possibility of better renal function and a restoration to a nearly normal quality of life. Numerous ESRD symptoms can be relieved by the transplanted kidney's ability to efficiently filter waste materials from the blood and preserve fluid and electrolyte balance.

Dialysis, which can be physically and time-consuming for patients, is also avoided by transplantation. Dialysis can have a big influence on a person's daily schedule since it requires frequent trips to a dialysis facility or the use of home dialysis equipment. Following a successful kidney transplant, patients can return to a more normal lifestyle and are no longer dependent on dialysis.

Furthermore, a kidney transplant that is successful can greatly increase a patient's longevity. Although PKD is a genetic disorder and cysts may develop in the transplanted kidney in the future, the disease usually progresses more slowly in donated kidneys than in native kidneys. This increases the likelihood that people with PKD will live long, healthy lives.

Moreover, kidney transplantation has a favourable effect on mental and emotional health in addition to physical health. A patient's overall quality of life can be considerably enhanced by the respite from the difficulties of dialysis, the restoration of kidney function, and the capacity to lead a normal life. It provides the chance to resume employment, form deep connections, and follow one's own ambitions.

The Risks and Considerations of Kidney Transplantation:

Although there are many advantages to kidney transplantation, it's vital to be aware of any possible risks and consequences. Being a major procedure, transplantation entails certain dangers, like bleeding, infection, and anesthesia-related side effects.

There's also a chance that the immune system of the receiver will reject the transplanted kidney. Patients need to take immunosuppressive drugs to avoid this, as they lower the risk of rejection by suppressing the immune system. But these drugs also make you more vulnerable to infections and other possible side effects like diabetes, high blood pressure, and bone damage.

After kidney transplantation, routine monitoring and follow-up care are crucial to early detection of any problems or rejection symptoms. Regular blood tests and clinical evaluations are usually performed on patients to guarantee the continued health and functionality of their transplanted kidney.

Conclusion:

A glimmer of hope is provided by kidney transplantation for PKD patients who have advanced renal illness. It offers the chance to swap out unhealthy kidneys for healthy ones, restoring renal function and enhancing general health and wellness. Ongoing monitoring, thorough assessment, and preparation are crucial because transplantation has some hazards. People with PKD are better equipped to choose their course of therapy by knowing the indications for kidney transplantation and the associated risks and benefits.

The Kidney Transplant Evaluation Process for Polycystic Kidney Disease

Making the decision to receive a kidney transplant is serious, particularly for people who have polycystic kidney disease (PKD). I have helped numerous PKD patients through this path as a physician and health and wellness coach, giving them the knowledge and encouragement they need to make an educated choice. I'll take you through the kidney transplant evaluation process for post-ketotic kidney disease (PKD) in this subchapter, outlining its many facets and potential roadblocks.

A thorough medical evaluation is the first step in the kidney transplant evaluation procedure. This entails a comprehensive review of the patient's medical history, taking into account any allergies, chronic illnesses, and prior procedures. It is critical to evaluate the disease's severity and effect on kidney function in people with Parkinson's disease (PKD). Typically, blood tests are used to determine the glomerular filtration rate and assess creatinine levels (GFR). An ultrasound or CT scan is another imaging test used to assess the quantity and size of kidney cysts.

A psychosocial examination is just as important as evaluating the patient's physical condition. The mental and emotional health of an individual can be greatly impacted by having a chronic illness such as Parkinson's disease (PKD). As such, assessing the patient's psychological well-being, support network, and transplant preparation is essential. This evaluation, which is typically conducted through questionnaires and interviews, aids in identifying any potential obstacles or worries that might surface throughout the transplant procedure.

Finding a qualified donor is one of the most difficult tasks in the evaluation process for kidney transplants for individuals with

Parkinson's disease. In contrast to other kidney illnesses, familial members are more likely to be suitable donors because PKD is frequently a genetic illness. Finding a suitable donor, however, can be difficult even within families because of things like blood type, tissue compatibility, and general health. Under such circumstances, transplant centres might look into matched exchange programmes or add the patient to a waiting list for deceased donors.

The evaluation process for kidney transplants heavily relies on transplant centres. A team of medical experts from these specialist clinics, including social workers, psychologists, nephrologists, and transplant surgeons, collaborate to make sure the patients receive all-encompassing care and support. At these centres, the coordinators act as a liaison between the patient and the medical staff, assisting them with all aspects of the evaluation procedure and answering any queries or worries that may come up.

The patient's medical and psychosocial history is typically discussed, and the kidney transplant procedure is thoroughly explained, during the initial consultation with the transplantation team. The patient has the chance to ask questions and get any doubts they may have answered during this time. The group will also talk about the advantages and disadvantages of transplantation as well as alternate forms of care like dialysis.

A number of examinations and screenings are carried out when the patient chooses to move on with the kidney transplant evaluation. These examinations aid in assessing the patient's general health and transplant eligibility. In order to assess the patient's heart, lungs, and other organs, the medical examination usually consists of blood and urine tests, chest X-rays, electrocardiograms, and consultations with many specialists. In order to gain further knowledge on pre- and post-transplant care, the patient could also participate in a transplant education programme.

The psychosocial assessment is a crucial part of the examination. This entails scheduling an appointment with a social worker or psychologist to evaluate the patient's mental and emotional preparedness for transplant surgery. To make sure the patient has the tools and coping processes needed to manage the stress of transplantation, problems like depression, anxiety, and social support are assessed. To detect any potential obstacles to the transplant process, the transplant team may also evaluate the patient's insurance coverage and financial situation.

The transplant team analyses the findings and decides if the patient is a good candidate for a kidney transplant after all required examinations and tests are finished. The decision is made in light of various considerations, including psychological preparedness, compatibility with possible donors, and general health. The patient may choose to locate a living donor or is put on the transplant waiting list if they are found to be a compatible match.

For PKD patients, the evaluation process for a kidney transplant is a difficult and complicated one. It necessitates a thorough evaluation of the patient's psychosocial and medical circumstances. Transplant centres and coordinators play a critical role in helping patients through this procedure by providing guidance and assistance. We enable people with Parkinson's disease (PKD) to make educated decisions about their health and the potential for a kidney transplant to give them a new lease on life by offering a road map and resolving any worries or obstacles.

Potential Challenges and Considerations in Kidney Transplantation for Polycystic Kidney Disease

Patients with Polycystic Kidney Disease (PKD) have a number of special difficulties and factors that must be taken into account while undergoing kidney transplantation. I have direct experience with the nuances and difficulties associated with managing Parkinson's disease (PKD) and navigating the transplantation process as a medical practitioner and health and wellness coach who focuses on holistic healthcare and wellness.

Kidney cysts filled with fluid are a characteristic of the genetic disease known as PKD. Over time, these cysts expand progressively, causing functional impairment and renal enlargement. The kidneys may eventually stop working, in which case a kidney transplant would be required. However, there are possible difficulties that people with PKD may have even following a successful transplantation.

The effect of PKD on transplant outcomes is one of the main obstacles. People with PKD may have a higher risk of complications and a lower long-term survival rate than people with other forms of kidney disease because of the underlying genetic causes and structural abnormalities linked to the disease. Research indicates that in comparison to those without non-cystic kidney disease, patients with PKD who have kidney transplantation may have increased incidence of surgical complications, graft rejection, and infection.

Furthermore, PKD may present as recurrent cysts in the kidney that has been transplanted. As PKD is a hereditary illness affecting the entire body, the kidney transplant may cause the cystic phenotype to resurface. This can make it difficult to manage the cysts, stop additional kidney damage, and guarantee the transplanted organ's long-term viability. As a result, careful observation and monitoring are necessary to identify cyst recurrences early and implement the necessary countermeasures to avoid consequences.

For those with PKD who have had kidney transplants, post-transplant monitoring and care are essential to maximising results. To keep an eye on the condition and functionality of the transplanted kidney, routine follow-up appointments are required. These appointments include imaging examinations, laboratory testing, and assessments of renal function. Lifestyle changes including maintaining a nutritious diet, getting regular exercise, and controlling stress can also improve general health and lengthen the life of a kidney transplant.

Some of these difficulties have been addressed by the notable progress made in the field of PKD transplantation in recent years. Better post-transplant care, more effective immunosuppressive drugs, and improved surgical methods have all improved the prognosis for those with PKD. It's vital to remember that every person has a unique experience, and that's why tailored care and management techniques are essential to meeting their individual demands.

Studies have indicated that there can be variation in the kind and degree of cyst involvement in PKD, which can affect the outcome of transplants. Therefore, prior to transplantation, a thorough assessment of the native kidneys' structural anomalies and cystic burden is crucial. This assessment can assist in identifying patients who might benefit from extra procedures, such as removing the native kidneys at the time of transplantation, or a nephrectomy.

Moreover, research has indicated that the existence of extrarenal PKD symptoms, including cerebral aneurysms or liver cysts, may affect the prognosis of transplant recipients. For complete therapy of their condition, patients with PKD who have extrarenal signs may need multidisciplinary care from experts in several specialties, such as neurology or hepatology.

In conclusion, kidney transplantation presents particular difficulties and factors for those with PKD. It is crucial to remember the effects of PKD on transplant results, the possibility of recurrent cysts in the kidney that was transplanted, and the significance of post-transplant monitoring and care. As a physician and health and wellness coach, I stress the need of managing Parkinson's disease (PKD) holistically, which includes individualised treatment plans, lifestyle changes, and interdisciplinary teamwork. Individuals with PKD can attain the best possible results and lead happy, full lives after transplantation by being aware of and taking action against these obstacles.

Post-Transplant Care and Management for Polycystic Kidney Disease

A crucial stage of a PKD patient's journey is post-transplant care. Following a kidney transplant, it is imperative to take a holistic approach to preserving the new organ's health and functionality. This calls for a trifecta of critical lifestyle adjustments, frequent monitoring, and medication therapies.

The use of immunosuppressive medicines is a critical component of post-transplant treatment. These drugs are essential in keeping the body from rejecting the kidney transplant. They lessen the possibility that the immune system will attack the new organ as a foreign body by inhibiting it. For the transplant to be successful over the long term, individuals with PKD must closely comply to their prescribed immunosuppressive treatment regimen.

It is critical to recognise that immunosuppressive drugs have a unique set of dangers and possible adverse effects. I collaborate closely with my patients as a physician and health and wellness coach to inform them of these dangers and provide them with the tools they need to make decisions about their care. I provide them all the information they need to assess the advantages and disadvantages of immunosuppressive drugs, including information on possible adverse effects.

Another essential component of post-transplant care is routine monitoring. Patients must see their transplant team for follow-up appointments on a regular basis following a kidney transplant. During these visits, several procedures such as imaging scans and blood tests are performed to evaluate the kidney transplant's functionality and overall health. Frequent monitoring makes it possible for us to identify early warning indicators of rejection or other issues, allowing for timely intervention and treatment.

After a kidney transplant, lifestyle changes are essential for long-term success in addition to medical measures. I collaborate extensively with my patients to assist them in putting into practise the required dietary adjustments, exercise regimens, and stress-reduction strategies. These changes are intended to enhance general wellbeing and support the kidney transplant's overall health and functionality.

Studies have indicated that a diet high in fruits, vegetables, whole grains, and lean proteins can improve the results of a transplant. Together, my patients and I develop customised meal plans that satisfy their unique dietary requirements and tastes and supply the essential nutrients to maintain their general health. In order to support renal function, I also stress the value of hydration and advise my patients to consume a sufficient amount of water each day.

Another essential part of post-transplant treatment is exercise. Frequent exercise has been demonstrated to enhance mood and general well-being, support weight management, and improve cardiovascular health. I collaborate with my patients to create customised workout regimens that suit their needs and tastes. Exercises including swimming, yoga, walking, and strength training may fall under this category. My patients can enhance their general level of fitness and encourage the best possible functioning of their transplanted kidney by adding exercise to their regular regimen.

Post-transplant care also requires the use of stress management strategies. For patients, the time after a kidney transplant can be emotionally and psychologically taxing. Stress levels can rise as a result of managing the effects of the transplant on daily life, adjusting to new drugs, and overcoming the fear of rejection. I work with my patients to teach them different stress-reduction methods, such mindfulness, meditation, and deep breathing exercises. My patients can effectively control their stress and enhance their general well-being by implementing these approaches into their daily life.

In conclusion, for PKD patients hoping to succeed long-term following a kidney transplant, post-transplant care and treatment is essential. Immunosuppressive drugs, frequent monitoring, and lifestyle adjustments are all part of the process. Patients with kidney transplant rejection syndrome (PKD) can enhance their overall quality of life and support the health and function of their donated kidney by closely following their recommended drug regimen, getting regular monitoring, and making the required lifestyle modifications. I'm dedicated to helping my patients through this process and giving them the tools they need to take control of their post-transplant care as a medical professional and health and wellness coach.

Chapter 17: Polycystic Kidney Disease and Personal Empowerment

Self-Advocacy in Polycystic Kidney Disease

Self-advocacy is essential for controlling Parkinson's disease. It enables people to actively engage in their own care and regain control over their health. An essential component of self-advocacy is effective communication. It is critical that people with Parkinson's disease (PKD) speak to their healthcare team in an effective manner about their needs, problems, and goals. This may entail stating preferences and priorities as well as seeking clarity and raising issues. People can make sure that their healthcare staff is aware of their particular situation and can adjust their treatment plan by being explicit about their requirements and goals.

Making informed decisions is yet another crucial component of PKD self-advocacy. People must have a complete awareness of their disease, available treatments, and any possible dangers or advantages. With the right information, patients can actively engage in the decision-making process and collaborate with their medical team to create a personalised treatment plan that meets their objectives and values. This could entail looking at various treatment choices, getting second opinions, and analysing the benefits and drawbacks of each choice. In the end, each person has the ability to make decisions based on their own knowledge.

For PKD patients to actively engage in healthcare decision-making and treatment planning, this is also essential. Patients should make an effort to interact, communicate, and ask questions of their healthcare staff so that their treatment plan is customised to meet their individual requirements and preferences. This may entail debating treatment objectives, looking into complementary therapies, and actively contributing to the creation of an all-encompassing care plan. Engaging in active involvement enables people to take charge of their health and guarantees that their opinions are acknowledged at every stage of the healing process.

In PKD, self-advocacy extends beyond choices made regarding medical care. It also includes a range of lifestyle adjustments and self-care practises. Proactive measures can be taken by people with PKD to control their illness and enhance their general wellbeing. This can entail taking up a nutritious diet, working out frequently, controlling stress, getting enough rest, and abstaining from dangerous drugs. By doing these things, people can take charge of things that can affect how their condition develops and improve their quality of life.

Moreover, self-advocacy in Parkinson's disease (PKD) include psychological well-being. An individual's mental health may suffer when they have a chronic illness such as Parkinson's disease (PKD). It's critical that people ask for help from their loved ones as well as from their medical staff. The emotional and psychological components of having Parkinson's disease (PKD) can be effectively managed with the use of counselling and psychology-related techniques. Individuals can acquire coping mechanisms and build resilience in the face of their condition's obstacles through therapy.

It is crucial to create a thorough self-care strategy in order to support oneself during the PKD management process. Every element of one's emotional, mental, and physical health should be included in this strategy. Individuals can lay a strong foundation for their health and well-being by making an investment in self-care.

To sum up, self-advocacy is essential to the treatment of Parkinson's disease. People with Parkinson's disease (PKD) can take charge of their health and well-being by actively participating in healthcare decisions, communicating effectively, and making educated decisions. Self-advocacy guarantees that each person's particular requirements and preferences are taken into account while enabling them to confidently navigate their healthcare journey. It is an effective tool that can improve overall healthcare and wellness and change what it's like to live with Parkinson's disease (PKD).

Self-Care Practices for Polycystic Kidney Disease

Stress Reduction Techniques

Your general and physical health may suffer as a result of stress. Stress management is especially crucial for those with PKD because it can worsen symptoms and cause problems. Thankfully, there are a number of stress-reduction strategies that can ease the load and encourage serenity and relaxation.

Deep breathing exercises are one useful method for reducing stress. Taking calm, deep breaths and concentrating on your breathing are the basic steps of this exercise. You lower your blood pressure and heart rate and trigger the body's natural relaxation response by doing this. Even a short daily session of deep breathing techniques can dramatically lower stress levels and foster inner calm.

Meditating is another helpful stress-reduction strategy. The goal of meditation is to clear your mind of the constant flow of ideas that fuel tension and anxiety. Regular meditation practise can help you become more observant of your surroundings and improve your capacity to react calmly and clearly to stressful situations.

Healthy Lifestyle Choices

The secret to controlling PKD and averting more issues is to maintain a healthy lifestyle. Making educated decisions about your food, exercise regimen, and sleeping habits can have a big impact on your general health and quality of life.

An important aspect of managing PKD is diet. Maintaining a low-sodium diet is crucial since too much salt can exacerbate renal function and cause fluid retention. For those with PKD, a diet high in fruits, vegetables, whole grains, and lean proteins is advised. Limiting your consumption of processed meals and sugary drinks is also advised because they might cause weight gain and renal strain.

Exercise on a regular basis is also essential for those with PKD. Moderate activity, like cycling, swimming, or walking, can help you maintain a healthy weight, strengthen and condition your body overall, and improve your cardiovascular health. Before beginning any fitness programme, you should, however, speak with your healthcare professional because your specific condition may need modifying some of the routines.

Another essential component of a healthy lifestyle is getting adequate sleep. Aim for seven to eight hours of good sleep every night to promote overall health and kidney function at its best. To encourage restful sleep, set up a soothing nighttime ritual, make your bedroom cosy, and stay away from stimulating activities and coffee right before bed.

Engaging in Activities that Bring Joy and Fulfillment

A vital component of self-care is making time for oneself and doing things that make you happy and fulfilled, especially for those with chronic illnesses like Parkinson's disease (PKD). Prioritizing the things that make you happy and give you a sense of purpose might help you feel better mentally and emotionally overall.

Investigate pastimes or artistic endeavours that provide you the chance to express yourself and follow your passions. Find hobbies or pastimes that bring you delight and a sense of achievement, such as gardening, writing, drawing, or playing an instrument.

Furthermore, maintaining relationships with friends and family can be a huge source of emotional support. As you navigate your PKD path, surround yourself with people you love and who understand you. It can be beneficial to share your feelings and experiences with others, and having them around can be consoling when things are hard.

Including methods of relaxation that promote overall well-being, such taking long baths, engaging in mindfulness exercises, or indulging in a favourite activity, can be quite beneficial. Engage in relaxing and rejuvenating activities for yourself since these times of self-care are crucial for handling the mental and physical strains of having Parkinson's disease.

Recall that practising self-care is a continuous process that calls for commitment and regularity. You can improve your general well-being and manage Parkinson's disease (PKD) by implementing stress reduction techniques, adopting a healthy lifestyle, and participating in activities that make you happy and fulfilled. Making your mental, emotional, and physical well-being a priority will improve all facets of your life as a sign of self-love.

Be gentle with yourself and give yourself room to manoeuvre as you set out on your self-care path. Each person's journey towards self-care is distinct, so it's critical to pay attention to your body and modify routines as necessary. Seek help from healthcare specialists who can provide specialised advice and support tailored to your individual needs, such as myself and my team of experts.

Never forget that you are not travelling through PKD alone. By adopting appropriate self-care techniques and building a robust support network, you can become an expert in handling your polycystic kidney disease and lead a happy, healthy life.

Cultivating a Positive Mindset in Polycystic Kidney Disease

Your physical and mental health may suffer as a result of PKD, just like with any other chronic illness. Realizing how much your mentality affects how you manage the illness is crucial. You can empower yourself to take on obstacles head-on and improve the quality of your life in general by intentionally deciding to adopt a positive mindset.

Practicing thankfulness has proven to be a very beneficial strategy for treating Parkinson's disease. Having gratitude in our lives helps us to see the good things in our lives instead of the bad things. A thankfulness practise has been linked to increased optimism, lower stress levels, and better mental health, according to research. You may change your perspective and find joy in the present moment even in the face of challenges by setting aside some time each day to think on the things you have to be thankful for.

A good mentality can also be developed by incorporating positive affirmations into your everyday practise. Phrases that support your goals, values, and positive attributes about yourself are known as positive affirmations. Rewiring your brain to accept empowering ideas and beliefs is possible if you repeatedly repeat these affirmations. You could say things like, "I have the ability to thrive despite my disability," or "I am strong and tough." It's important to remember your innate strength and resilience when handling post-ketotic diarrhoea (PKD), and you can do this by deliberately selecting these affirmations.

A useful method to change your viewpoint and improve your general well-being is to reframe unfavourable thoughts. Particularly for someone managing a chronic illness like PKD, negative thoughts can be fairly prevalent. But by rephrasing these unfavourable ideas, you can turn failures into chances for improvement and put your attention on the good things in your life. For example, you can choose to reframe a setback, such a decline in kidney function, as a beneficial lesson that will help you manage and take better care of yourself.

A positive outlook is essential for developing resilience, which is something that is necessary for managing Parkinson's disease (PKD). The capacity to pick oneself up after failure and adjust to changing conditions is resilience. That makes it possible for you to stay positive and persistent in the face of difficulties. Self-care alternative and complementary strategies are a good strategy to build resilience. Physical, emotional, and spiritual well-being are all included in these approaches for holistic well-being. The resilience and positive outlook that you cultivate can be greatly enhanced by practising yoga, meditation, deep breathing techniques, and mindfulness.

Asking for help from family, friends, medical professionals, and support groups is another essential part of developing a positive outlook. It can greatly aid in the management of Parkinson's disease (PKD) to be surrounded by people who share your experience and who can offer advice, support, and understanding. You can find a sense of community and support by discussing your worries and experiences with people who are facing like difficulties, which validates your own struggles. Healthcare experts like me can also help you overcome the challenges of controlling Parkinson's disease (PKD) by providing you with specialised guidance and solutions.

Developing a positive outlook is a valuable strategy for managing Parkinson's disease (PKD) that can improve your general health and give you the strength to overcome obstacles with hope and fortitude. You may change your viewpoint and discover delight in the here and now by engaging in gratitude practises, repeating positive affirmations, and rephrasing unfavourable ideas. It also helps you better negotiate the challenges of managing Parkinson's disease (PKD) when you combine alternative and complementary self-care practises and ask for help from family and support groups. You have the power to choose optimism, so remember that you can design a plan for effective PKD management by intentionally choosing positivity.

Setting Goals and Celebrating Milestones in Polycystic Kidney Disease

I've had the honour of dealing with many individuals who are managing and coping with polycystic kidney disease as a medical practitioner and health and wellness coach (PKD). Based on my personal experience, I have realised the significant influence that goal-setting and commemorating achievements can have on the process of efficiently managing post-ketotic kidney disease.

Establishing objectives gives our actions and decisions direction and purpose, acting as a roadmap. Having specific goals in mind can be quite motivating when it comes to managing a chronic condition such as Parkinson's disease (PKD). These objectives might be short- or long-term, and they must be time-bound, relevant, quantifiable, reachable, and specified (SMART).

It's critical to first decide what you want to accomplish. This could involve enhancing renal function, lessening pain and suffering, controlling lifestyle elements like nutrition and exercise, or even attending to your mental health. Once your objectives have been determined, divide them into more manageable, smaller steps.

For instance, if improving kidney function is your main objective, you can start by concentrating on preserving a healthy blood pressure or making dietary adjustments like cutting back on sodium. Greater goals become more achievable and less daunting when they are divided into smaller, manageable steps.

Setting goals requires keeping track of your progress. There are several ways to accomplish this, including journaling, using apps on smartphones, or even wearing wearables that monitor health information. You may evaluate what is functioning well and make the required adjustments along the road by routinely reviewing your progress.

Recognizing accomplishments is just as vital. No matter how little the milestone, celebrating it gives you a sense of success and inspires you to keep working hard. Acknowledge and treat yourself when you reach a goal or get closer to one. This might be as easy as rewarding yourself with a pat on the back, getting yourself something nice, or even telling loved ones about your accomplishments so they can encourage and support you.

It is crucial to consider the motivations behind your goals in order to generate a feeling of purpose and drive. What motivates you to properly manage your PKD? Is it to make your life better, support the people you love, or achieve your own goals? Understanding your core driving forces will help you maintain concentration and dedication to your objectives, particularly under trying circumstances.

The advantages of including a healthcare team in goal-setting and milestone celebrations should also be noted. As a health and wellness coach, I collaborate with a group of professionals from various health and wellness domains to offer my patients all-encompassing care. All facets of controlling Parkinson's disease (PKD) are taken care of thanks to this interdisciplinary approach, which includes food regimens, coping mechanisms, psychological support, and lifestyle changes.

Setting goals and celebrating achievements can be made even more effective by embracing complementary and alternative approaches. These methods include self-care exercises like yoga, acupuncture, mindfulness, and meditation, among others. By fostering emotional and mental well-being in addition to physical well-being, these techniques create a more comprehensive approach to controlling Parkinson's disease.

In summary, goal-setting and commemorating achievements are essential components of PKD management. They offer guidance, meaning, and inspiration in addition to facilitating introspection and acknowledging individual accomplishments. People with PKD can go through life with more confidence and resilience if they follow a step-by-step approach, work with a healthcare team, and embrace complementary and alternative therapies. Keep in mind that you have a complete team of professionals at your disposal who are ready to help and mentor you as you work toward your objectives and celebrate each victory along the road. You are not alone on this trip.

Chapter 18: Polycystic Kidney Disease and Financial Considerations

Understanding the Financial Impact of Polycystic Kidney Disease

It is critical to realise that PKD is a chronic illness that needs ongoing medical supervision. The expense of diagnosis, which entails a number of tests and imaging investigations, is where the financial burden starts. Certain tests, including CT scans and ultrasounds, can be highly costly, particularly for those without comprehensive health insurance. Furthermore, to identify the precise genetic mutation causing PKD and validate the diagnosis, genetic testing might be required. The financial burden these exams place on individuals and their families may increase.

Upon confirmation of the PKD diagnosis, attention turns to controlling the disease's symptoms and complications. Drugs are essential for managing pain, combating infections, and regulating blood pressure. But these drugs can be expensive, particularly when you take into account that people with PKD frequently need to take them for a long time. Since not all prescriptions may be fully covered, the financial impact of prescription costs can be especially difficult for people who depend on government assistance programmes or do not have access to good health insurance.

To properly treat their disease, people with PKD may need to undergo a variety of medical procedures in addition to medication. For example, big cysts that cause pain or discomfort may require cyst aspiration or drainage. These treatments can be costly, and the total outlay may be too much if they must be done repeatedly. In a similar vein, patients with more severe cases of Parkinson's disease (PKD) can need kidney transplantation or cyst decortication. The financial consequences of these treatments are significant and include hospital stays, surgeon fees, and post-operative care costs.

Making changes to one's lifestyle is another crucial component of successful PKD management. These adjustments frequently entail eating differently and exercising frequently, both of which can significantly improve a person's general health and wellbeing. Regretfully, there may be financial implications associated with leading a healthy lifestyle. The cost of fresh produce, lean meats, and fresh fruits can often be higher than that of processed foods. Monthly costs may also rise for workout equipment or gym subscriptions. People with Parkinson's disease (PKD) and their families need to know how these lifestyle changes will affect their finances and figure out how to adjust their spending plans.

For people and families coping with the financial effects of Parkinson's disease, being able to estimate and manage spending is essential. It is imperative to develop a thorough budget that accounts for all medical costs, including prescription drugs, surgery, and doctor visits. The possibility of variations in these costs must also be taken into account, since the degree and course of Parkinson's disease might change over time. Some of the financial strain can be reduced by budgeting for unforeseen medical expenses like ER visits or hospital stays.

Managing the financial implications of Parkinson's disease (PKD) requires navigating the intricate healthcare system and making use of all available options. Seeking advice from a social worker or financial counsellor is advised, as they can offer insight into possible grants, financial aid programmes, or nonprofits that might help defray some of the expenses. Numerous pharmaceutical companies also provide patient assistance programmes that allow qualifying persons to receive medication at no cost or at a reduced cost. Investigating these choices can have a big impact on how the financial burden of PKD is managed.

In summary, PKD can significantly affect a person's and their family's financial situation in addition to being a medical hardship. The money spent on prescription drugs, medical treatment, and lifestyle adjustments may mount up rapidly, so budgeting for them demands forethought and creativity. Individuals and their families can more skillfully handle the financial problems by being aware of the financial implications of Parkinson's disease (PKD), planning and managing their spending, and investigating all available options. Recall that you have assistance to help you manage the financial effects of PKD and that you are not alone on this path.

Insurance Options for Polycystic Kidney Disease

Insurance plays a crucial role in the management of any chronic condition, and PKD is no different. I have direct experience with the difficulties PKD patients encounter in getting the insurance coverage required for their treatments and drugs because I work as a holistic healthcare physician and health and wellness coach.

Private insurance is among the most popular kind of insurance that people can get. PKD patients should carefully study the facts of their private insurance plan because there are considerable variations in the coverage and cost of these plans. This entails knowing what the copayments and deductibles are, what treatments and medications are covered, and whether there are any limitations or restrictions on coverage.

Many PKD sufferers may be eligible for government programmes like Medicare and Medicaid in addition to private insurance. Medicare is a government health insurance programme that mostly provides coverage to people 65 years of age and older, as well as people with specific disabilities. Conversely, Medicaid is a combined federal-state programme that offers low-income individuals and families health coverage.

It's critical that people with Parkinson's disease (PKD) comprehend the eligibility standards and specifics of these programmes' coverage. Medicare Part A provides hospital stays, skilled nursing facility care, and certain home healthcare services; on the other hand, Part B includes outpatient care, doctor visits, and certain preventative services. Prescription drugs are covered under Part D.

State-by-state variations exist in Medicaid coverage and qualifying standards. Generally speaking, Medicaid pays for a large number of medical services, such as doctor visits, hospital stays, prescription drugs, and long-term care. Additional services, such dentistry and vision care, might be provided by certain governments.

Although navigating the insurance system can be difficult, there are tools available to support patients with Parkinson's disease in understanding their rights and coverage alternatives. One such resource is the PKD Foundation, a nonprofit that offers assistance and information to those with PKD. Among the many services provided by the foundation is a helpline manned by qualified experts who can address queries and issues pertaining to insurance.

The National Kidney Foundation is a valuable resource that provides information and assistance to those with kidney illness. In addition to financial aid programmes and advice on navigating the insurance system, the foundation offers resources on insurance options.

Knowing what is covered is only the first step; in order to guarantee they get the drugs and treatments they require, people with Parkinson's disease (PKD) also need to be their own advocates. To handle denials or restrictions on coverage, this may entail corresponding with pharmacy benefit managers, insurance companies, and healthcare providers. Advocating for the best possible care and navigating the insurance system can be made easier with a solid support structure, such a care team.

Patients with Parkinson's disease (PKD) can reduce the financial burden of their illness by learning about and utilising insurance options. Investigating prescription assistance programs—such as those provided by pharmaceutical companies—that could give qualified people free or heavily discounted drugs is one way to do this. Moreover, generic pharmaceuticals may be less expensive than name-brand ones.

Moreover, lifestyle changes may be very helpful in controlling Parkinson's disease (PKD) and possibly lowering medical expenses. Maintaining overall kidney health involves avoiding tobacco and excessive alcohol usage, managing stress, exercising regularly, and adopting a nutritious diet. High blood pressure and kidney stones are two PKD problems that these lifestyle choices can help avoid or control.

Finally, insurance choices play a vital role in the management of polycystic kidney disease. Patients with Parkinson's disease (PKD) need to be aware of their private insurance policies, look into government programmes like Medicare and Medicaid, and be strong advocates for themselves to make sure they get the drugs and treatments they need. Patients suffering with Parkinson's disease (PKD) can enhance their quality of life and efficiently manage their disease by comprehending their coverage options, navigating the insurance system, and taking action to reduce the financial burden of their condition.

Financial Assistance Programs for Polycystic Kidney Disease

Patient Assistance Programs:

Patient assistance programmes are intended to help patients who cannot pay the costs of their treatments and medications by providing financial support. Usually provided by pharmaceutical firms, these initiatives are designed to assist individuals with particular medical illnesses, such as Parkinson's disease (PKD).

Patients with Parkinson's disease (PKD) may be eligible for the "Patient Assistance Program" offered by the PKD Foundation. A variety of PKD-related charges are covered by this programme, such as prescription drug prices, medical equipment costs, and travel fees to and from doctor's visits.

Patients who are uninsured or underinsured and who can demonstrate financial need are among the qualifying requirements that must be met in order to apply for this programme. Medical documents, proof of income, and other pertinent data may need to be submitted as part of the application process.

Charitable Organizations:

Patients with Parkinson's disease (PKD) can receive financial support from charitable groups in addition to patient assistance programmes. These organisations frequently have funds or programmes specifically designed to assist people with Parkinson's disease (PKD) and their families. Typically, they receive funding from grants and contributions.

The American Kidney Fund (AKF) is one such group that offers financial aid for medical costs, such as prescription drug costs, travel expenditures to and from dialysis sessions, and health insurance premiums. The "Helping Individual Patients" initiative of the AKF is intended especially to support people with chronic kidney disease, particularly PKD.

People with PKD diagnoses and household incomes that fit the program's requirements annually are among the requirements that must be met for eligibility. Usually, the application process include providing proof of income, health records, and other pertinent data.

Other Resources:

To lessen the financial strain of managing PKD, there are more options available in addition to patient support programmes and philanthropic organisations. These resources could be nonprofit groups that offer services and financial support to people with long-term illnesses, as well as government aid programmes and local resources.

The Social Security Disability Insurance (SSDI) programme is one such tool; it offers monthly financial payments to those with impairments, including those who have Parkinson's disease (PKD). In order to be eligible for SSDI, a person must have paid payroll taxes into the Social Security system and have a disability that keeps them from working. The application procedure might be difficult, and it might call for further proof of impairment in addition to medical records.

The State Health Insurance Assistance Program (SHIP) is an additional resource that offers Medicare beneficiaries—including those with PKD—free, individualised counselling and support. Counselors at SHIP may assist people with navigating the Medicare system, comprehending their options for coverage, and locating resources and programmes that can save money.

In addition, PKD sufferers may be eligible for financial aid or support services from local, regional, or national organisations or foundations. These organisations might offer grants, scholarships, or other financial aid to assist in paying for medical bills, travel expenditures, or other demands related to the disease's management.

It is crucial that PKD patients and their families actively look for and investigate these services and financial aid programmes. For information on the particular services offered in your area, I strongly advise you to get in touch with social workers, patient advocacy organisations, and your healthcare professionals. They can guide you through the application process, offer support and direction, and make sure you are taking advantage of all the resources and financial aid that are available to you.

Recall that treating PKD involves more than just changing one's diet and way of living. It also involves controlling the disease's financial effects. You may lessen the financial burden of PKD and concentrate on what really matters—your health and well-being—by making use of the financial aid programmes and resources that are available to you.

I hope you found this subchapter useful in learning about the financial aid options available to those with Parkinson's disease. We shall examine how diet and nutrition play a part in managing Parkinson's disease (PKD) in the upcoming chapter. Watch this space for helpful hints and recommendations on optimising your diet for optimum kidney health.

Financial Planning for Polycystic Kidney Disease

1. Importance of Budgeting:

Making a budget is essential to manage your money, particularly if you have a chronic condition like PKD. You can clearly see your income, expenses, and areas where you may save money by making a budget. Make a note of every source of income you have, including investments, salaries, and any disability benefits you could be eligible for. Next, keep a tab on all of your out-of-pocket costs, such as prescription drugs, medical bills, dietary supplements, and any necessary lifestyle changes. It's crucial to be meticulous and account for even the smallest costs, including the cost of driving to doctor appointments or over-the-counter drugs.

Find areas where you might be able to reduce expenses after you have a clear view of your income and outlays. Seek methods to cut back on wasteful spending, such eating out or overspending on entertainment. To obtain the greatest offers, think about searching for generic drugs or comparing costs at other pharmacies. You can more efficiently arrange finances and make sure you have adequate resources to handle your PKD-related expenses by practising cautious budgeting.

2. Saving for Medical Expenses:

Continuous medical treatment is necessary for polycystic kidney disease, including routine blood work, imaging scans, doctor visits, and maybe operations. If these medical costs are not budgeted for in advance, they can mount up quickly and cause a large financial strain. It is essential to establish a savings strategy expressly for your PKD-related medical costs.

To begin, determine about how much you would require for each area of your healthcare. Find out how much typical consultations, lab work, prescription drugs, procedures, and any other condition-specific treatments will cost. Decide on a savings target after you have a ballpark estimate. Ascertain the monthly amount that you can reasonably save, and open a different savings account that is only used for your medical costs.

Set up an automated transfer from your paycheck or checking account to your special medical savings account to help you automate your savings. In this manner, you'll be able to gradually accumulate a financial cushion to lessen the impact of medical bills and won't have to rely on remembering to save regularly. Furthermore, look into your employer's health savings account and flexible spending account alternatives. These can help you save money expressly for medical bills and have tax benefits.

3. Exploring Long-Term Financial Options:

When living with PKD, it's critical to investigate long-term financial choices that can offer further help in addition to budgeting and saving. Here are some crucial things to remember:

- Benefits for Disability: You can qualify for disability benefits based on the severity of your Parkinson's disease and how it affects your capacity to work. Find out what your nation or region's requirements are for receiving disability payments and how to apply for them. Speak with a financial advisor or an expert in disability benefits so they can help you through the process and make sure you get the most out of the benefits that are available.

- Insurance Coverage: Examine your current insurance coverage, such as your life, health, and disability plans. Ascertain that the coverage you have meets your unique demands. Recognize the terms and conditions of your coverage, taking into account any PKD-related restrictions or exclusions. To obtain the greatest coverage for your needs, compare insurance plans or providers if necessary.

- Estate Planning: Estate planning is an important part of your long-term financial well-being, even though it's not a topic you usually associate with managing a chronic condition. Creating the required legal documents, such as wills, trusts, and powers of attorney, is estate planning. In the event that you die away or become unable of making decisions, these agreements serve as a roadmap for the distribution of your assets and express your preferences. Having an estate plan in place can bring you piece of mind and guarantee that your loved ones are taken care of in the future, even though it might not have a direct impact on your day-to-day financial management.

Recall that financial planning is a continuous process that needs to be carefully monitored and adjusted as your situation does. Make sure your long-term financial plans, savings objectives, and budget are all in line with your present needs and objectives by reviewing them on a regular basis. Seek expert advice from a financial advisor or planner who is familiar with the particular difficulties involved in managing a chronic disease. You can concentrate on your health and well-being without experiencing unnecessary financial stress when you have a thorough financial plan in place.

We shall explore the significance of self-care strategies for PKD management in the upcoming chapter. When dealing with a chronic illness like Parkinson's disease (PKD), self-care is an essential part of holistic health and can have a big impact on your general wellbeing. Stay tuned as we discuss different self-care strategies to assist you deal with the difficulties of having Parkinson's disease (PKD), such as stress reduction, relaxation methods, and exercise.

Chapter 19: Polycystic Kidney Disease and Relationships

Communicating About Polycystic Kidney Disease With Loved Ones

I have devoted my life to advocating for holistic health and wellness, so I am aware of how crucial good communication is to the management of a complicated illness like polycystic kidney disease (PKD). It is important to create a solid support network and promote understanding among your loved ones in addition to talking about symptoms and available treatments.

Receiving a PKD diagnosis can be very daunting. Acknowledging the fact that you have a chronic illness and navigating the challenges of disclosing it to the people who matter most to you are two very different things. It is normal to be nervous and uncertain about how to bring up the topic, but if you approach it with an honest and open mind, you may lay the groundwork for a network of people who will be understanding and supportive.

Adopting vulnerability is the first step towards successful communication regarding PKD. It is crucial to keep in mind that you are not alone on this trip. You provide your loved ones a space to offer support and understanding when you share your challenges, anxieties, and concerns with them. Talk to someone about your diagnosis, your symptoms, and how it affects your day-to-day activities. You are allowing your loved ones the chance to comprehend your circumstances and feel your pain by being honest and frank with them.

But it's also important to keep in mind that everyone handles emotions in a unique way. While some family members could find it difficult to accept the truth of your illness, others might be happy to help and understand. Setting limits and honouring each person's emotional journey are crucial when it comes to talking about your PKD. Tell your loved ones about any boundaries you have if there are specific subjects or conversations that make you feel anxious or uncomfortable. This will make it easier for them to comprehend your demands and guarantee that discussions about your health are constructive and encouraging.

Not only should you establish limits, but you also need to enlighten your loved ones about PKD. Building empathy and understanding requires education. Give a thorough explanation of PKD, including how it affects the kidneys and possible effects on the body as a whole. To assist your loved ones in understanding the complexities of the situation, share with them any pertinent study or information you have come across. Giving them information will make them more capable of helping you throughout your PKD journey.

Giving your loved ones support and understanding is just as vital as having an honest and open conversation about PKD. Recall that while they accept the diagnosis, they can be feeling a variety of emotions of their own. Invite them to share their thoughts and worries, and listen to them without passing judgement. You can provide a secure space for your loved ones to express any concerns or issues they may have regarding your condition by encouraging open lines of communication. By doing this, you not only make your relationship stronger but also guarantee that all parties involved feel heard and understood.

Giving your loved ones practical support is just as vital as having an open conversation and offering emotional support. A person with PKD may need to make several dietary and lifestyle adjustments. Share these changes with your family and friends, and provide them tools and resources to better understand your dietary requirements and constraints. By including them in your treatment plan and offering them helpful assistance, you foster a sense of solidarity and shared accountability for managing your Parkinson's disease.

It is certainly difficult to deal with a chronic illness such as Parkinson's disease (PKD), but you can make the journey easier if you and your loved ones can communicate well. Recall that candid discussions serve as the cornerstone of a robust support network. Establish limits as needed, enlighten your loved ones about PKD, and be there to support and understand them while they work through their feelings. You two can create a network of love and support that will support you as you deal with the highs and lows of having PKD.

Adjustments and Challenges in Relationships With Polycystic Kidney Disease

A person's relationships with loved ones are significantly impacted by a diagnosis of post-conception depression (PKD), in addition to the person's own life. The physical and emotional aspects of intimacy can be profoundly impacted by PKD symptoms and therapies. People with Parkinson's disease (PKD) frequently experience fatigue, pain, and diminished libido; these physical restrictions can cause tension in personal relationships. It is critical that people with PKD and their partners have honest and open communication about how the disease affects their sexual lives. This could entail looking into different intimate relationships, getting professional assistance, or lowering expectations to account for the disease's effects.

Moreover, PKD may cause problems in family dynamics. In addition to having a hereditary component, PKD can also impact family members. Those who have the illness may experience emotional strain and feelings of guilt as a result. One family member may be solely responsible for providing care in some situations, which could damage their bond with the affected person. For the sake of the patient's and their loved ones' wellbeing, it is critical to set up boundaries that are clear, maintain open lines of communication, and, when needed, seek outside assistance.

Moreover, PKD may affect social interactions. Isolation and social disengagement may result from the disease's physical and psychological burdens. Social isolation may be exacerbated in people with PKD by their fear of being judged or their sense of being misinterpreted by their peers. It's critical for people with PKD to build new social networks or seek out assistance from those who share their challenges. Participating in support groups, seeking treatment or counselling, or connecting with virtual communities can alleviate feelings of isolation and foster a feeling of inclusion.

Having the support of close ones and keeping up positive relationships are essential for coping with PKD's difficulties. On the other hand, it is typical for people with PKD to feel uncomfortable asking for assistance or burdening others with their problems. It's critical to communicate one's needs to loved ones and to appreciate the benefits of vulnerability. People and their loved ones can collaborate to develop workable answers and emotional support by exchanging experiences and worries.

In addition to depending on their close support network, people with PKD may find it helpful to consult a specialist. This may entail attending support groups led by medical professionals or engaging with therapists or counsellors who specialise in chronic illness. These channels offer a secure environment for exchanging stories, picking up tips from others, and acquiring coping mechanisms to deal with the difficulties of Parkinson's disease. Healthcare practitioners can also provide helpful guidance on how to handle stressful situations, establish self-care routines, and have challenging conversations with loved ones.

With PKD, self-care is essential for coping with the changes and difficulties it brings. It's critical that people put their mental and physical health first. This can involve eating a balanced diet, exercising frequently, practising mindfulness or relaxation techniques to reduce stress, and looking for hobbies or creative outlets. Making time for oneself improves one's capacity to actively participate in relationships with loved ones as well as one's general state of well-being.

In summary, PKD significantly affects the relationships that those who have the illness have with one another. Intimacy, family relationships, and social ties may all be impacted. Managing these difficulties requires open and honest communication, professional assistance when needed, and self-care as a top priority. In the end, maintaining supportive and healthy relationships can help people with Parkinson's disease (PKD) and their loved ones improve overall well-being by accepting the adjustments and challenges that the disease entails.

Supporting Loved Ones With Polycystic Kidney Disease

It can be devastating for both the patient and their family to learn that a loved one has Parkinson's disease (PKD). Because the illness is progressive and chronic, it calls for constant care and long-term management. It is imperative that caregivers approach their work with compassion and understanding. It's important to acknowledge that PKD can lead to weariness, mental turmoil, and physical discomfort in the person you're caring for.

The capacity to comprehend and experience another person's emotions is known as empathy, and it is an essential trait for caretakers. By showing empathy, you establish a judgment-free environment in which the individual with PKD can freely communicate their feelings and worries. They may feel heard and understood as a result, which is beneficial when they are coping with a chronic condition.

One of the most important caring skills is active listening. It entails keeping eye contact, focusing entirely on the speaker, and offering both verbal and nonverbal affirmation. Someone with Parkinson's disease (PKD) can freely express their ideas and experiences when you actively listen to them. They may feel less alone and more supported during their illness journey as a result.

For someone with PKD, practical help is just as important as emotional support. Your loved one may require assistance with everyday duties or activities connected to their health due to the physically taxing nature of both the disease's symptoms and treatment. This can involve helping with personal care, making appointments, managing medications, and providing transportation to doctor's appointments. You can lessen the load and support the person with PKD in maintaining their independence by providing them with useful assistance.

As you assist a loved one with Parkinson's disease, remember to take care of your own emotional health and needs as well. Given how demanding caring for a person with a chronic illness may be, caregiver burnout is a real possibility. Setting your emotional and physical wellness as a top priority will help you avoid burnout.

In order to maintain your own wellbeing while providing care for someone with Parkinson's disease, self-care is crucial. This can involve things like working out, practising meditation, keeping a journal, or taking up relaxing and joyful hobbies. It can also be helpful to take pauses, ask friends and family for help, and participate in fulfilling social interactions. Recall that you cannot serve from an empty cup, and that in order to properly care for your loved one, you must first take care of yourself.

Creating a support network is a crucial part of helping carers maintain their emotional health. Making connections with those who play a similar caring role can offer support and a sense of unity. Caretakers of people with Parkinson's disease (PKD) might benefit greatly from support groups designed especially for them, as they offer a platform for exchanging experiences and knowledge. Social media groups and online forums are additional tools for information and support.

It can be difficult to manage the emotional toll of taking care of a person who has a chronic illness. A wide range of emotions, such as grief, rage, frustration, and guilt, are natural. Managing these feelings is a crucial part of keeping your own mental health in check. To examine these emotions and create coping mechanisms, going to therapy or counselling can offer a secure setting.

In summary, helping family members with Parkinson's disease (PKD) calls for a blend of compassion, attentive hearing, and hands-on help. You may establish a secure environment for your loved one to communicate their emotions by offering emotional support and acknowledging their experiences. By providing useful support, you can lessen their physical stress and preserve their independence. To properly care for a loved one with PKD, you must also prioritise your own emotional well-being and engage in self-care. Recall that you are not travelling alone and that getting help from others can be quite beneficial.

Self-Care and Relationships in Polycystic Kidney Disease

Having devoted my professional life to advocating for holistic health and wellness, I am adamant that self-care is an essential part of treating polycystic kidney disease rather than only a luxury (PKD). In my work as a PKD patient care provider, I have personally witnessed how putting off self-care can result in emotional, relational, and physical difficulties. In this section, I hope to clarify the critical role that self-care plays in preserving wholesome relationships while managing Parkinson's disease (PKD) and offer doable methods for implementing it into your everyday routine.

People with post-traumatic stress disorder (PKD) frequently experience overwhelming feelings and tend to put their own needs last. But putting off self-care puts our relationships with loved ones at serious risk in addition to endangering our physical health. In order to foster and preserve good relationships, it is crucial to place a high priority on self-care and set appropriate boundaries.

Realizing the importance of setting boundaries is one of the first stages towards developing self-care. It's important to set boundaries for our physical and emotional capabilities when we have a chronic illness like PKD. This entails knowing when to say no and refraining from going over our own boundaries. We may safeguard our own wellbeing and make sure that those closest to us are aware of and accept our limits by establishing and effectively communicating boundaries.

Getting help is another crucial component of self-care for people with Parkinson's disease (PKD) who want to keep their relationships intact. People with Parkinson's disease frequently experience feelings of isolation and overwhelm due to the difficulties they encounter. But by putting ourselves out there and asking for help—from friends, family, or support groups—we not only learn more about our own conditions but often find comfort and validation in the company of others who are going through similar things. Seeking assistance can provide one a sense of relief and empowerment. Support can take many different forms, such as emotional, practical, or educational support.

Setting aside time for self-care practises that enhance general wellbeing is essential for controlling Parkinson's disease (PKD) and preserving wholesome relationships. It's critical to keep in mind that taking care of ourselves is an investment in our own wellbeing, not a selfish one. This can involve doing things like consistent exercise, practising mindful meditation, or taking up enjoyable hobbies. Not only can these activities enhance our physical well-being, but they also elevate our emotional state and facilitate more effective communication and interpersonal interactions. Prioritizing self-care enables us to be more completely present in our relationships, which in turn nurtures and fortifies those bonds.

Apart from these approaches, self-care also entails embracing coping mechanisms that facilitate our management of the distinct difficulties associated with having Parkinson's disease. Chronic illnesses such as Parkinson's disease (PKD) can frequently be erratic and cause changes in mood and state of health. We can better manage the ups and downs of our illness by learning coping mechanisms, such as engaging in stress-reduction exercises, getting professional treatment when necessary, and adopting an optimistic outlook. By encouraging resilience and adaptation, these coping mechanisms not only improve our individual wellbeing but also have a favourable effect on our interpersonal connections.

To sum up, self-care is essential to managing PKD and preserving wholesome relationships. We can better manage the complexities of our relationships by prioritising self-care activities, setting boundaries, and getting help. By doing these things for ourselves, we can also take care of our own well-being. Recall that taking care of ourselves is an essential investment in our pleasure and well-being, not selfishness. We are better able to support our loved ones and create enduring bonds when we take care of ourselves. Accept self-care as a crucial component of managing your Parkinson's disease and observe how your relationships grow and prosper.

Chapter 20: Polycystic Kidney Disease and the Future

Advances in Polycystic Kidney Disease Research

In my capacity as a physician and health and wellness coach, I am always researching the most recent findings and advancements in the field of polycystic kidney disease (PKD). We will explore the fascinating field of PKD research in this subchapter, talking about possible discoveries, new therapeutic approaches, and how patient engagement will influence PKD management going forward.

Let's pause to consider the path that PKD research has gone over the years before delving into the most current developments. The world's scientists and researchers have worked tirelessly to improve our understanding and treatment of this complicated illness.

In the past, PKD was discovered in the early 20th century, but the genetic cause of the illness was not discovered until the 1980s. Thanks to developments in DNA sequencing technology, scientists have been able to pinpoint the mutations that cause most cases of autosomal dominant PKD in particular genes, like PKD1 and PKD2 (ADPKD).

Since then, scientists have been working harder to understand the fundamental causes of Parkinson's disease (PKD) and create novel therapeutic approaches. The significance of cellular signalling pathways in the course of Parkinson's disease (PKD) is one area that has attracted a lot of study.

A increasing amount of data in recent years has suggested that PKD development and progression are significantly influenced by the deregulation of specific signalling pathways, including the mTOR pathway. Because of this information, mTOR inhibitors are being investigated as possible PKD treatments.

Everolimus is one such mTOR inhibitor that has demonstrated potential. Everolimus has been shown in clinical trials to be an effective means of preventing kidney cyst formation in ADPKD patients, therefore protecting their kidney function. This discovery has given sufferers and medical professionals alike fresh hope because it presents a focused strategy for controlling the progression of Parkinson's disease.

Researchers have also been examining the potential of alternative therapeutic drugs, such as vasopressin receptor antagonists, in addition to mTOR inhibitors. Vasopressin is a hormone that increases fluid output, which in turn encourages the creation of kidney cysts. These antagonists can lessen the formation of cysts and delay the course of the disease by preventing vasopressin from doing its job.

Vasopressin receptor antagonists, such tolvaptan, have shown encouraging outcomes in clinical trials. These medications have been linked to a delayed deterioration in renal function in addition to being demonstrated to reduce the volume of kidney cysts. Given that the advantages of these treatments are greatest in the early stages of the disease, these findings are significant because they highlight the significance of early intervention in the management of Parkinson's disease.

Even if these pharmaceutical treatments have a lot of potential, it's critical to understand the value of managing PKD holistically. When combined with medical therapies, lifestyle changes and self-care routines can greatly enhance the general wellbeing of persons with Parkinson's disease (PKD).

Recent research has demonstrated the advantages of consistent exercise and a nutritious diet in the management of Parkinson's disease (PKD). Exercise has been demonstrated to enhance cardiovascular health, which is important for PKD patients, and to slow the growth of kidney cysts. Including mindfulness- and relaxation-promoting exercises like yoga and tai chi can also help lessen the psychological toll that comes with having a chronic illness.

Diet is also very important in managing Parkinson's disease. A diet low in protein and salt may help prevent kidney cyst formation and maintain renal function, according to research. Furthermore, a number of dietary supplements, including antioxidants and omega-3 fatty acids, have demonstrated potential in lowering oxidative stress and inflammation, two factors linked to the advancement of Parkinson's disease.

Beyond these changes in lifestyle, patient empowerment and involvement will play a critical role in determining how PKD is managed in the future. Patients actively participate in their own healthcare journeys and are more than just beneficiaries of medical care. Patients can actively participate in research studies, advocate for their needs, and actively engage in self-care behaviours to help discover new treatment options and improve those that already exist.

Numerous patient-led groups are committed to raising awareness of PKD and providing support, research, and resources. These groups give patients and their families a forum to interact, exchange stories, and take an active part in advocacy and fundraising initiatives. Patients may strengthen their voices and have an impact on decision-makers, researchers, and healthcare professionals by banding together as a collective force.

To sum up, PKD research has advanced significantly in recent years, revealing possible discoveries and new avenues for treatment. To enhance the quality of life for people with Parkinson's disease (PKD), researchers are devoting their time and energy to investigating cellular signalling networks and creating tailored pharmaceutical interventions.

But it's crucial to keep in mind that patient participation and holistic healthcare are essential elements of successful PKD management. We can improve the well-being of patients with Parkinson's disease (PKD) and open the door for more promising developments in PKD research and treatment by implementing lifestyle changes, self-care routines, and patient empowerment.

I'm dedicated to being on the front edge of PKD research as a physician and health and wellness coach, and I pass this knowledge forward to my patients. By working together, we can overcome the challenges posed by Parkinson's disease and enable people to take charge of their health, resulting in a more satisfying life.

The Importance of Hope and Resilience in Polycystic Kidney Disease

It's common to feel overwhelmed, demoralised, and powerless while dealing with a chronic condition like polycystic kidney disease (PKD). The effects on day-to-day living, the physical symptoms, and the uncertainty about the future can all be detrimental to one's mental and emotional health. It's important to keep in mind, too, that resilience and hope can be quite helpful in coping with the difficulties presented by PKD and preserving optimism.

One should never undervalue the power of an optimistic outlook. Studies have indicated that maintaining a happy outlook can significantly influence both our mental and physical well-being. It can strengthen our defences against illness, lower our stress levels, and even make it easier for us to handle hardship. It can be especially difficult, although not impossible, for those with PKD to keep an optimistic outlook.

Gratitude is a discipline that can help you develop a positive outlook. We can change our perspective and discover joy in the present by concentrating on the things for which we are thankful, despite hardship. Reframing our attitudes and cultivating optimism and hope can be achieved by journaling our appreciation or by just pausing each day for a few minutes to consider the benefits in our life.

Having a solid support network is another important strategy for building resilience. Having friends, family, and medical professionals who are sympathetic to the struggles faced by someone with Parkinson's disease (PKD) can be quite beneficial. These people can foster a feeling of community and belonging by offering emotional support, useful assistance, and a listening ear.

Studies have also demonstrated that social support enhances the capacity to manage chronic illness and enhances health outcomes. In order to manage post-ketotic depression (PKD), it can be helpful to have someone to share the journey with, lean on at difficult times, and celebrate achievements with. For people with Parkinson's disease (PKD), locating a support system—through social networks, online forums, or personal relationships—can be a lifesaver.

In addition to recognising the possibility of a better future through continued research and breakthroughs in therapy, developing a strong support network and maintaining an optimistic outlook are critical components of managing Parkinson's disease (PKD). Recent years have seen tremendous developments in PKD research, including improvements in treatment options, diagnostic methods, and possible solutions.

To better understand the fundamental causes of Parkinson's disease (PKD) and create tailored medicines that will decrease the disease's progression, scientists and medical professionals are working nonstop. Gene treatments, novel pharmaceuticals, and other cutting-edge techniques are being tested in clinical trials. The quality of life for persons who have PKD can be significantly enhanced, and these developments give hope for a future in which the disease's effects can be reduced.

Furthermore, more accurate PKD management and monitoring are now possible because to technological improvements. Diagnoses can now be made earlier and with greater accuracy thanks to advancements in imaging techniques like computerised tomography (CT) scans and magnetic resonance imaging (MRI). Early intervention, including the adoption of lifestyle changes and treatment regimens, can halt the disease's progression as a result of early discovery.

For people with Parkinson's disease, tailored treatment is also coming soon. Researchers are finding particular gene mutations linked to various disease forms because to developments in genetic testing. This discovery opens the door to customised care plans and therapies that take into consideration each patient's particular genetic makeup.

Overall results can be improved and treatment effectiveness can be maximised with this customised strategy.

It is critical that people with PKD and those who support them remain up to date on the most recent findings in the field of medicine. Acquiring this knowledge can instil a feeling of strength and optimism for the future. People can actively participate in their own care and increase our understanding of Parkinson's disease (PKD) by continuing to be involved with medical experts, advocacy groups, and research institutes.

To sum up, hope and fortitude are critical for overcoming the difficulties associated with Parkinson's disease. Maintaining optimism and a sense of agency in the face of severe chronic illness requires developing a positive mindset, creating a strong support network, and keeping up to date on research and treatment developments. Through the acceptance of hope and adaptability, people with Parkinson's disease (PKD) can travel through life with more courage, strength, and resolve, which will ultimately improve everyone's quality of life and future.

Advocacy and Awareness in Polycystic Kidney Disease

In the management and treatment of any chronic condition, but particularly in the case of polycystic kidney disease, advocacy is essential (PKD). As a physician and a health and wellness coach, I have personally witnessed the transformative effects of community support and advocacy on the quality of life for people with Parkinson's disease. Through my work with the PKD community and other patient advocacy organisations, I have seen firsthand the transforming power of creating awareness and encouraging a feeling of group action.

For those with PKD, patient advocacy groups like the National Kidney Foundation and the PKD Foundation are vital sources of support. These groups put up a lot of effort to spread knowledge about the illness, offer educational materials, support research projects, and support laws that assist people with PKD. In order to guarantee that patients' needs are met and their rights are upheld, they work to give patients' voices more weight.

It's important to spread knowledge about PKD for a number of reasons. Primarily, it aids in clearing up misunderstandings regarding the illness. Many people lack empathy and compassion because they are uninformed of the prevalence and effects of Parkinson's disease (PKD). We can enlighten the public and eliminate the stigma attached to PKD by raising awareness. Consequently, this cultivates an atmosphere that is more encouraging and welcoming for both patients and their family.

Moreover, PKD awareness campaigns promote early diagnosis and identification. Being a progressive condition, PKD frequently goes undiagnosed until later on, when symptoms worsen. We can encourage people to seek medical assistance sooner by raising awareness of the condition and educating them about its symptoms, which may result in early intervention and better outcomes.

Potentially more financing and research is another advantage of increasing awareness. Compared to more common disorders, PKD, like many other uncommon diseases, frequently receives less money and attention. But greater knowledge also means more money being spent on R&D by the public and private sectors. This may result in ground-breaking findings and improvements in PKD patients' treatment alternatives.

Organizing people into groups is a great way to push for change. We can strengthen our voices, create networks of support, and have a bigger effect by uniting as a community. The annual PKD Awareness Day, which is observed on September 4th, is one instance of this. People come together from all over the world on this day to promote awareness about PKD through a variety of events and activities. Collective efforts to raise awareness and advocate for change include social media campaigns, fundraising walks, educational seminars, and community gatherings.

Advocacy and raised awareness have a profound effect. Patients and their families gain from it, but the healthcare system as a whole also gains from it. By promoting early intervention and preventive measures, we can lessen the demand on healthcare resources by increasing awareness about Parkinson's disease (PKD). Moreover, raised awareness can result in quicker and more precise diagnoses, which enables medical professionals to create individualised treatment programmes that are tailored to the particular requirements of each patient.

Public policy and healthcare activities are significantly shaped by advocacy and awareness. We can guarantee that the requirements of the PKD community are acknowledged and taken care of at the policy level by fighting for increased financing for PKD research, better patient access to care, and the inclusion of PKD in public health initiatives. The combined voices of caregivers, patients, and medical professionals have the ability to improve the state of healthcare.

To sum up, in the management and treatment of polycystic kidney disease, advocacy and awareness are critical. Patient advocacy organisations play an essential role in providing patients with assistance by amplifying their voices and lobbying on their behalf. Clearing the air about PKD is crucial for eradicating myths, promoting early detection, and securing funds and research. The lives of people with PKD and the larger healthcare system can be significantly improved by the PKD community working together. Together, we can create a future in which PKD is more effectively recognised, treated, and eventually cured.

Living Well With Polycystic Kidney Disease

Sometimes it feels impossible to manage a chronic illness like polycystic kidney disease (PKD). A person's physical and mental health may suffer as a result of the daily struggles, the long-term uncertainty, and the ongoing need for alertness. However, this does not have to be the case. It is possible to live well with PKD and have a fulfilling life if you adopt the correct strategy and mindset.

Taking care of oneself is crucial to living well with Parkinson's disease. Your primary concern should be taking care of yourself. Meeting your requirements for physical, emotional, and mental wellness entails doing this. It is crucial to pay attention to your body's needs and provide it with the necessary rest and nutrients. Self-care includes taking part in enjoyable activities, learning relaxing techniques, and taking care of your relationships.

Setting up a healthy lifestyle as a top priority is essential for maintaining physical health. This entails implementing a nutritious diet, exercising frequently, and getting adequate rest. Your kidney function and general health can be supported by eating a diet high in fruits, vegetables, whole grains, and lean proteins. Limiting your consumption of salt, sugar-filled beverages, and processed foods is also crucial. Exercise routines like yoga, swimming, or walking can not only improve your physical health but also lower stress and enhance your mental health. Furthermore, in order for your body to heal and rejuvenate, you must make sure you obtain adequate restorative sleep.

Another essential component of living well with Parkinson's disease is keeping an optimistic mindset. When dealing with a chronic illness, it is normal to feel a range of emotions. However, it is crucial to have an optimistic outlook and learn coping mechanisms for the difficulties that lie ahead. Having a strong support system of family and friends around you might be a great way to get understanding and encouragement. To help manage the emotional aspects of living with Parkinson's disease (PKD), seeking therapy or joining support groups can be beneficial. Keep in mind that you have resources at your disposal to support your survival and that you are not travelling this path alone.

It's also critical to acknowledge that managing PKD may necessitate making certain lifestyle adjustments. This can mean modifying your everyday schedule, arranging modifications to your workplace, and coming up with efficient stress-reduction strategies. You can manage the responsibilities of having a chronic illness by learning to set limits and prioritise your needs. It's critical to let your loved ones, the medical staff, and your employers know about your requirements and restrictions so they can provide you with the support and understanding you need.

You might investigate complementary and alternative therapies in addition to conventional medical treatments to enhance your general health and wellbeing. Acupuncture, massage therapy, meditation, and herbal supplements are a few examples. Participating in these therapies under the supervision of a licenced healthcare provider can offer extra assistance and alleviation from PKD-related symptoms.

Living with Parkinson's disease (PKD) can be difficult, but it's crucial to keep in mind that you have the ability to manage your health and lead a happy life. You may overcome the difficulties and thrive with PKD by putting self-care first, leading a healthy lifestyle, keeping a positive mindset, and asking for help when necessary.

We have discussed the significance of good lifestyle choices, self-care, and keeping an optimistic mindset when living with Parkinson's disease (PKD) in this chapter. Your physical, emotional, and mental well-being must come first. You should also ask for help from your loved ones, the community, and your healthcare team. You may preserve your general health and well-being and lead a full life by taking the required actions to take care of yourself and manage the problems that come with Parkinson's disease (PKD). Recall that your courage and perseverance in the face of difficulty define you, not your condition.

Milton Keynes UK
Ingram Content Group UK Ltd.
UKHW020247221123
432980UK00016B/923

9 798223 802662